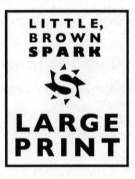

LITTLE,
BROWN
SPARK

LARGE
PRINT

BRAIN WASH

Detox Your Mind for Clearer Thinking, Deeper Relationships, and Lasting Happiness

DAVID PERLMUTTER, MD, and AUSTIN PERLMUTTER, MD

WITH KRISTIN LOBERG

LITTLE, BROWN **SPARK**

LARGE PRINT EDITION

Copyright © 2020 by David Perlmutter, MD, and Austin Perlmutter, MD

Hachette Book Group supports the right to free expression and the value of copyright. The purpose of copyright is to encourage writers and artists to produce the creative works that enrich our culture.

The scanning, uploading, and distribution of this book without permission is a theft of the author's intellectual property. If you would like permission to use material from the book (other than for review purposes), please contact permissions@hbgusa.com. Thank you for your support of the author's rights.

Little, Brown Spark
Hachette Book Group
1290 Avenue of the Americas, New York, NY 10104
littlebrownspark.com

First Edition: January 2020

Little, Brown Spark is an imprint of Little, Brown and Company, a division of Hachette Book Group, Inc. The Little, Brown Spark name and logo are trademarks of Hachette Book Group, Inc.

The publisher is not responsible for websites (or their content) that are not owned by the publisher.

The Hachette Speakers Bureau provides a wide range of authors for speaking events. To find out more, go to hachettespeakersbureau.com or call (866) 376-6591.

ISBN 978-0-316-45332-5 (hardcover) / 978-0-316-42639-8 (large print)

LCCN 2019946529

10 9 8 7 6 5 4 3 2 1

LSC-C

Printed in the United States of America

For everyone seeking reconnection

Contents

Contents

PART II
BREAKING THE SPELL

BRAIN WASH

Introduction

A New Reality

If you want to be happy, be.

—Leo Tolstoy

When was the last time you felt truly happy, fulfilled, clear-minded, well rested, and deeply connected not only to yourself but also to the people and world around you? If it's been a while, this book is for you. You're far from alone in this feeling. Millions of people are suffering today and either don't realize it or don't know what to do about it. Some have given up and are going through the daily motions as best they can. It doesn't have to be this way.

You can wake up from this state of monotony and start pursuing lasting joy and a deeply meaningful existence — even as you move through struggles, disappointments, and challenges. Those are inevitable. What is not inevitable is feeling chronically untethered, foggy-minded, anxious about an uncertain future, and frustrated—maybe even shattered—by life itself. The thing is, there are very real ways to avoid many of these feelings and, even more important, create ongoing happiness in your life. Some of the strategies shared in the pages ahead will be easier than others, but all will be doable and accessible.

Let us confess from the get-go: we haven't attained a perfect realization of this goal. We're on this journey with you. Our belief is that we've found a powerful way to reframe and reclaim our potential for exceptional mental and physical health, and we can't wait for you to implement this in your own life.

Here's the paradox that persecutes us today: modernity provides us with infinite opportunities. We can eat whatever we want whenever we want. We can completely immerse ourselves in the vast, enticing world of digital media. We can buy goods and services and even find potential mates with the touch of a button or swipe of a finger. We can live around the clock in a virtual world where everything about us is public, from our thoughts and perspectives to our purchases, photos, browsing habits, likes and dislikes, and location. We think this 24-7 "new reality" should make us healthy and happy. But it doesn't. The systems in place to meet—and exceed in many regards—all our basic needs do not create Utopia. Quite the opposite. We struggle with soaring rates of largely preventable illnesses, and many of us are more lonely, depressed, and anxious than ever before. Genuine joy remains elusive.

The crazy thing is, despite what the incessant news cycle would have us believe, our modern world is relatively peaceful. Yet poll a large, diverse group of people and the vast majority of them will say they think we live in perilous times. They are fearful, uneasy, and nervous. They feel trapped. Life, overall, is just not a pleasant experience. What's more, distrust in one another has reached a new high. A 2014 survey of ten thousand Americans revealed the biggest division in political ideologies in decades, and since 2004, the percentage of people with negative views of the opposing party has more than doubled.[1] For anyone keeping abreast of the news, this finding is probably not surprising.

We promise to bring you a new framework for living your life. Together we are going to find a way to cultivate and maintain a more fulfilling existence beyond robust health and psychological well-being. It's time for a brain wash of an entirely different kind.

THE PROMISE ... AND THE PROBLEM

Imagine for a moment that you're not particularly concerned about anything. You feel grounded and energetic, not the least bit worn, weighed down, burned out, or dead inside. You trust your body's innate physiology to take care of you and heal on its own. You're not overly stressed because you have confidence that any challenges you have will work themselves out. You're comfortable not knowing what tomorrow will bring, though you have a sense of positive agency over the possibilities. And you are okay with the past, however traumatic it was. You're even okay with friends who have completely different viewpoints from yours. Everything feels right. Your private self-talk is hopeful, relaxed, and open. The sound track of your life is a song you want to play over and over again.

It's hard to consider this level of calmness and contentment when the obligations of the modern world feel more inescapable and crushing with each passing day. But this can be your reality. The secret is knowing what's going on in your head and then changing the circuitry that leads you down destructive paths. This book builds from a simple premise:

Our brain's performance is being gravely manipulated, resulting in behaviors that leave us more lonely, anxious, depressed, distrustful, illness-prone, and overweight than ever before. At the same time, we feel disconnected from ourselves, from others, and from the world at large.

Few people would debate the fact that poor choices in our day-to-day activities influence our health. For example, we know that junk foods are bad for us and, over time, can lead to all manner of diseases. So why is it that we persist in eating these foods? Why do we consistently choose to consume the wrong things? The answer is complicated, but part of the solution is to understand a basic truth: we are being programmed to ingest these poisons.

Our dietary choices are among many lifestyle habits that can lead to either wellness or chronic disease. Chronic disease accounts for 70 percent of American deaths: half of Americans are suffering from at least one chronic illness, including diabetes, heart disease, cancer, and Alzheimer's disease.[2] And while we continue to argue over how to change our health-care system, we forget that we spend 75 percent of our health-care dollars on preventable diseases.[3] The World Health Organization now ranks chronic degenerative diseases such as the illnesses we just mentioned as collectively the number one cause of death on the planet, ahead of famine, infectious diseases, and wars.[4]

That may not be news to you if you are aware of the critical link between poor diet and disease. But what you may not realize is that **the food you eat and the beverages you drink change your emotions, your thoughts, and the way you perceive the world.** Just as important, your mood and perceptions also directly and powerfully influence your dietary choices. This fact is exploited by the food-production industry and creates a vicious cycle that will destroy your health—and your mind. We will show you how to break it. But this is so much bigger than just our food choices.

Through incessant exposure to advertisements, you are being reminded thousands of times a day that instant gratification is the way to happiness. The message comes in subliminally. Billions of dollars are spent to persuade you to keep pursuing happiness the wrong way, by literally rewiring your brain so that you crave the things that bring you further from your goal. You might think that you are doing everything you are supposed to do in order to succeed at life, but still, things are not wonderful. Social media tells you that everyone else is having a great time. Ads tell you that buying something will change your life or that a diet pill will instantly fix your love handles. Your attempts at eating healthfully are thwarted by a limitless supply of delicious and cheap calories. You feel like being unhealthy is *your fault.* This depressing scenario is now the norm, fueling a culture of chronic stress. Unfortunately, this type of stress is toxic to the brain, damaging the very parts of it that help you have a sense of agency—to feel in control of your life. And in your attempts to cope, you again turn to instant gratification, making it harder to break the neural circuits that trigger and reinforce this behavior. The escape hatch moves further away. In the chapters ahead, you'll discover exactly how this happens and what you can do about it. **You can be better.** Your body and mind want to improve, they just need to know how.

From a biological perspective, many factors lead us into the trap of instant gratification. We'll explain these factors over the course of the book. For example, you may already know that chronic inflammation is closely linked to many of the diseases that afflict us today. But you may not know that chronic inflammation also influences the brain—leading you to make poor decisions and act impulsively.

In part 1, "Living Under the Influence," we'll reveal the mental hijacking that undermines each and every one of us in our search for meaning, joy, and lasting wellness. In part 2, "Breaking the Spell," we'll present the tools necessary to think more clearly, strengthen bonds with others, and develop healthful habits. For those of you who need a structural blueprint, we've got a practical ten-day program that puts all the strategies together. Indeed, you can begin to change the trajectory of your health and life in ten days.

WHERE WE COME FROM

It's not every day that you read a book written by a father and son. We joined forces from two completely different generations sharing one question: What makes health and happiness so elusive? Below, we talk about where we're coming from in our own individual words.

Austin: While completing my residency in internal

medicine, I followed the traditional approach to health, which emphasizes the diagnosis and treatment of individual diseases. I did my best to properly identify and manage my patients' many problems. Yet despite my efforts, most of my patients seemed less than interested in adhering to my carefully crafted plans. Why would they decide against taking life-prolonging medications or eating a diet that would, in theory, protect them from developing heart failure or diabetes?

I mistakenly believed that my interests and those of my patients were the same. This failure of reasoning was resolved when I started asking my patients one question: What do you really care about? I expected my patients to tell me that their health was paramount, but I was shocked by how wrong my assumption turned out to be. Very few people told me that their health was their priority, at least not in the way I expected. Instead, what they valued most were their families, friends, and, surprisingly, even their hobbies. It became clear that these were the things that brought them meaning and joy. What they really cared about was *connection*. Good health was simply a tool to get them there.

I realized I needed to reframe my perspective on how to help others. If I truly wanted to assist my patients in the best way possible, I needed to start with connection.

This led me to deepen my understanding of how we interact with ourselves, with others, and with our environment. I saw that meaningful connection was not found by buying new things or engaging in quick digital interactions. And yet our culture seems increasingly set on directing us to pursue these endeavors. Worrisome data show that we spend an increasing amount of time each day focused on the short-term fix and miss out on the very moments that consistently improve the quality of our lives. I now understand that the question is not just how to foster connection but also how to identify and remove the aspects of life that keep us from experiencing it. I started by looking at how to improve connection and found that escaping from disconnection may be even more important. The chance to explore this critical topic with my father and to bring these findings to the world has been one of the most gratifying experiences of my life.

David: My mission over the past four decades has been to do my very best to empower through knowledge. The way in which lifestyle—including diet and physical activity—relates to health and longevity has always been a central theme in my books and lectures. I've been presenting this information because it might not otherwise be obvious in the face of rampant advertising. It has become clear to me that disconnection is at the core of what's keeping us from truly embracing health, longevity, happiness, and contentment. These goals are attainable.

This book has been a labor of love. What an honor it is to have been given the opportunity to connect with my son on this project and learn from his perspective as an individual as well as a representative of his generation. This gives me great hope in looking to the future.

UNWIRE AND REWIRE YOUR BRAIN FOR THE BETTER

When we began to research this book, we could not have predicted what we would find. Within the first month, both of us felt at once alarmed and transformed as we embraced the importance of our task. The further we dug into the research, the more we knew we were onto something *big*—something that had the potential to affect not only individuals (including us) but also the planet and its societies as a whole. This is not a trivial point. The destiny of Earth is at stake here. That may sound like an overstatement, but we will make our case. Happy, connected people make for a happy planet, both in the context of individual health and the environment's health. When you look around you and consider the state of our planet, you know that things are currently not sustainable. **We need you.** And we need one another.

We fully appreciate the significant benefits that come from living in the modern world. And we're not advocating that you remove yourself from it. For example, when it comes to modern technology, we couldn't have written this book without online research databases and video conference calls. Instead, we are calling for a different approach to our digital world, one in which we are conscious users of our technology—not used by it. Our world provides incredible opportunities to learn from and connect with one another through digital networks, but it's imperative that we use these opportunities the right way. The world has so much to offer, and the tools to change your life—and health—are right in front of you. We can't wait to share them.

Despite the scope of this book, our strategy focuses on creating a practical framework that you can implement in your life right away. We live and work in the modern world and understand the limitations of what's possible and realistic. The good news is that so much of what's keeping us from achieving lasting health and happiness is within our power to change. We know you can get there—through an overhaul of your mind's operating system. We don't have to be victims of poor health, loneliness, and the constant urge to pursue the next short-term fix. This new framework—a reconnecting, life-changing "brain wash"—teaches you how to clean up your mind and activate the brain pathways that bring clear thinking, deep relationships, and mental well-being.

Ready? Let's get to work.

PART I

LIVING UNDER THE INFLUENCE

CHAPTER 1

Disconnection Syndrome

A Sad State of Affairs

In the materialistic way of life, there's no concept of friendship, no concept of love, just work, twenty-four hours a day, like a machine. So in modern society, we eventually also become part of that large moving machine.

—His Holiness the 14th Dalai Lama, *The Book of Joy*

When you woke up this morning, what was the first thing you did? What sequence of events describes your typical morning? Our bet is that your routine has shifted dramatically from what it was just ten or fifteen years ago. How many minutes go by before you check your cell phone or scroll through media, social or otherwise? How many swipes and clicks do you perform? What do you normally eat for breakfast? Cold cereal, a bagel, muffin, pastry, or a doughnut on the go? What kinds of personal interactions do you have with your loved ones before you leave the house?

As you drive to work on the same route you've always taken, are you tuned in to yourself and calmly focused on the day ahead? Or are you feeling anxious, scattered, and overwhelmed? Are you texting, checking your email, and talking on your cell phone while you should be concentrating on the traffic signals? When you arrive at work, do you find it hard to focus and concentrate for long stretches of time without the pull of digital distractions? Do you eat lunch at your desk? Do you multitask throughout the day with your phone always nearby? Do you connect with people mostly through emails, texts, and phone calls rather than in person?

After work, do you make time for a refreshing outdoor walk or workout? Or do you get home, pour yourself a drink, and eat dinner — perhaps a meal consisting of processed or packaged food? Do you find yourself going to bed exhausted and spent from the day yet unable to sleep? Do you wake up intermittently throughout the night? And when you rise in the morning, do you wake up feeling down and out, only to go through the same monotonous routine again?

Our society has experienced a fundamental shift since the beginning of the twenty-first century, largely because of an explosion in the availability of personal technology that keeps us locked on the grid. It's estimated that 70 percent of humans on the planet now own a smartphone.[1] Data show that the average internet user spends more than two hours a day on social networking.[2] One survey found that 42 percent of the time Americans are awake, their eyes are fixated on a television, smartphone, computer, tablet, or other device.[3] Supposing the average American sleeps eight hours a night, that means people spend about six hours and forty-three minutes a day staring at a screen. Over the course of a typical life span, that's 7,956 days, or nearly twenty-two years.

This tectonic shift has led to a culture of disconnection all around us—we walk around with our heads down, fixated on our devices, avoiding ideas that differ from our own, while confronting constant messages telling us what to do (eat more, buy more, post more, be "liked" more). If we're really paying attention, we can feel it within us. A void. A sense of longing. Participating in our modern consumerist existence is physically changing our brains. How, exactly? It is cutting off access to the highly evolved part of the brain that lets us see the big picture and make well-thought-out decisions. Simultaneously, it is strengthening the pathways that make us impulsive, anxious, fearful, and constantly craving a quick fix. This rewiring leads us to spend our time and money on things that do not bring us long-term happiness. It leaves us constantly unsatisfied. And that's exactly where corporate interests want us to be, because it leads to higher profits. The frightening truth is this: our brains are increasingly running on a program controlled by others—namely, commercial interests hoping to capture the primitive brain's desire for instant gratification.

Your attention and your decisions are sold to the highest bidder, to companies with the best understanding of how to manipulate your psychology and biology for their own profit. These companies understand how to tap into powerful neurological pathways, creating a nearly irresistible addiction to short-term pleasures and a commercialized illusion of sustainable joy. We call this state of separation from sustainable happiness *disconnection syndrome*, and it's time to take a stand against it. Below is a visual representation of the top eight characteristics of disconnection syndrome. We'll be exploring each of these in detail within the context of brain health and function.

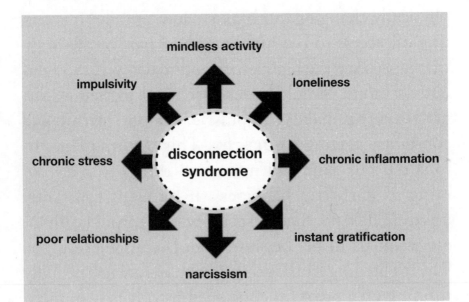

A MODERN-DAY PARADOX

Step 1 in taking a stand against disconnection syndrome is to take a hard look at the difference between the world we're led to believe in and the actual facts. Looking behind the curtain at the reality we currently face can be daunting. But through this process comes true power. By appreciating things for the way they are, you begin to take back control of your life. With an understanding of how and why your brain has been hijacked, you can choose to change your life. Replacing choices that don't help you with those that do frees you to pursue long-term satisfaction and lasting fulfillment. And when you can take control of your brain's wiring, you can build a system that continues to make those good choices.

At first glance, it would seem we've never had more opportunities to pursue and achieve happiness than we do today. Everyone on social media appears to be smiling, and TV commercials would have us believe there is a drug to fix every mood disorder we might experience. And yet rates of anxiety and depression continue to climb. Suicide rates increased in nearly every state from 1999 through 2016, and among adolescents, rates soared 56 percent between 2007 and 2016.[4] This is the case even though the number of antidepressant prescriptions in the United States has gone up by more than 400 percent since the 1990s.[5] And we're taking more drugs in general, both legal and illegal. Around half of older folks (age sixty-five and up) with anxiety are taking benzodiazepines (e.g., Xanax, Valium, and Ativan) — medications with well-known and potentially life-threatening side effects.[6] Insomnia afflicts about one-fourth of American adults, leading many to turn to sleep aids.[7] What's more, global trends show rates of alcohol use rising, especially in the increasingly Westernized economies of India and China.[8] Binge drinking among adolescents and young adults is also on the rise worldwide.[9] To be sure, these sobering statistics are not reflective of a satisfied culture.

One might expect that our obsessive use of social media would make us feel more connected to others, but nearly half of Americans report sometimes or always feeling lonely. People reporting this feeling at the highest rate are adults between the ages of eighteen and twenty-two.[10] In addition, only around half of Americans report having meaningful in-person social interactions.[11] Aristotle was right when he wrote "Man is by nature a social animal," but we need to get back to the way in which Aristotle socialized. We bet he didn't suffer from disconnection syndrome.

To understand the reasons for these modern problems — and the way to solve them — we must turn to the most powerful tool we have. The brain has been shaped by the mightiest force on earth: evolution. It has adapted to changing pressures over the course of several million years so that it can thrive under a variety of conditions. The more we know about its resiliency and plasticity, the more incredible it seems. But we need to understand that the brain, for all its brilliance, still runs programs written long ago that can be commandeered or "hacked" by modern technologies, much the way a computer virus can infect software and change its functionality. Our primal desire for sweet foods and our need for social acceptance, for example, made a lot of sense in millennia gone by, when we had to worry about the scarcity of food resources during winter or the possibility of exile from the tribe. **What were once valuable adaptations that helped us survive have now become entry points for exploitation.** These core survival systems have long been part of our brain's hardwiring, but they are now the targets of corporate efforts to manipulate your decision-making processes and capture your money, attention, and loyalty. Most important, we're losing our grasp of our sense of self and self-worth—our identities are under assault from the constant stream of messages telling us what we're supposed to look like, feel like, and strive for. We are left feeling inadequate. It's time to reconnect to our brains' higher levels of thinking and functioning.

> Your thoughts and decisions are at stake because they are valuable—they translate into corporate profit.

The human brain is an incredible gift of seemingly endless complexity and ability. One thing that makes humans special is our brains' disproportionately large *prefrontal cortex*, sitting just inside the front of our skulls and constituting nearly one-third of the neocortex—the most recently evolved part of the brain, which consists of gray matter surrounding the deeper white matter of the cerebrum. It is the prefrontal cortex that is credited with higher-order brain functions such as our ability to plan for the future, express empathy, see things from the point of view of another, make thoughtful decisions, and engage in positive social behavior—basically all the things that make us human. (By contrast, a chimpanzee's prefrontal cortex makes up just 17 percent of its neocortex, and a dog's comprises 13 percent.) The prefrontal cortex orchestrates thoughts and actions that help us achieve our goals, from simple objectives such as cooking a meal to complex tasks such as writing a book. The term for the activity carried out by the prefrontal cortex is *executive function*. Executive function includes the ability to differentiate among conflicting thoughts; determine good and bad, better and best, same and different; understand future consequences of current activities; work toward a defined goal; predict outcomes of actions based on past experience; and have social "control" (i.e., the ability to suppress urges that, if not contained, could lead to socially unacceptable outcomes). Scientific research on executive function is currently exploding and shows that, indeed, many environmental factors within our control can affect the health and functionality of the prefrontal cortex and ultimately our behavior and well-being.

Unfortunately, much of modern life conspires to keep our brains from taking full advantage of the prefrontal cortex. Instead, we find our actions driven by impulsivity, fear, and a need for instant gratification, which are triggered by overactivation of the *amygdala* (an emotional center of the brain) as well as by the constant stimulation of the brain's reward circuits (more on this shortly).

There is a way out of this mess. We'll reveal how improving your diet, sleep hygiene, exposure to nature, exercise habits, conscious consumption, mindful practices, and interpersonal interactions can affect your relationship with your own mind and help you reconnect to

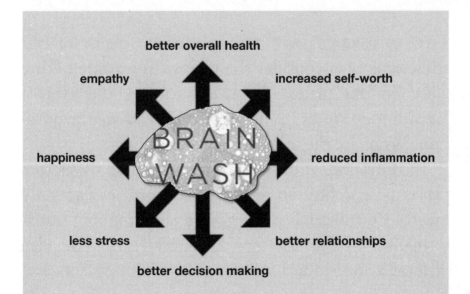

your prefrontal cortex, literally building a better brain, which leads to better decisions and, in the end, a better you. Here's a visual representation of what we'll be covering:

BIOLOGICAL WARFARE

> *Inevitably, the manufacturers of processed food argue that they have allowed us to become the people we want to be, fast and busy, no longer slaves to the stove. But in their hands, the salt, sugar, and fat they have used to propel this social transformation are not nutrients as much as weapons— weapons they deploy, certainly, to defeat their competitors but also to keep us coming back for more.*

> —MICHAEL MOSS, *SALT SUGAR FAT*

THE QUICKEST WAY TO GRASP the depth of our addictions is to consider the biological warfare taking place on our plates. We readily accept the idea of "health food stores," but that certainly raises the question: What are the other food stores selling?

In the world of nutrition, we've become slaves to a perverted redefinition of what the word *food* actually means. Our diet has undergone a jaw-dropping transformation in the last ten thousand years. The idea of food as nutrition has become a vanishing concept. Instead, we consume energy-dense, nutrient-poor foods and beverages that wreak havoc on our health, especially on our brain health. A surplus of calories pushes our bodies into a downward spiral of chronic, preventable diseases—including obesity, hypertension, heart disease, diabetes, and cancer—and, ultimately, to an early death. Research conducted by the Friedman School of Nutrition Science and Policy at Tufts University suggests that poor eating causes nearly *one thousand deaths each day* in the United States from heart disease, stroke, or diabetes.[12] The worst part? Consuming nutrient-poor foods forces the body and brain into a perpetual loop that keeps us craving and coming back for more, restructuring the brain for the worse. And this is getting costly: in 2016, the direct and indirect costs of chronic diseases resulting from obesity were $1.72 trillion.[13] That's almost 10 percent of the nation's gross domestic product.

Unfortunately, any person carrying around the extra weight caused by consuming empty calories is deemed a failure—rather than a victim of the toxic, addictive system that created this pathological state in the first place. If you're someone who has struggled with your weight, please understand that the deck has been and remains actively stacked against you and your willpower. *This is not your fault.* In chapter 7, we'll show how and why modern foods, which have been stripped of everything healthful, became so addictive and ever-enticing. The power of this addiction is not unlike that of addiction to hard-core drugs such as heroin and cocaine. We can draw many parallels between the opioid crisis and obesity epidemic. Craving painkillers is similar to craving sugar.

Sugar, ultraprocessed foods, and obesity are demonized daily. But maybe these are not issues for you. Perhaps you eat pretty well, would not consider yourself a junk-food addict, and remain at a healthy weight. Everyone comes to this book with varying strengths and weaknesses. For you, maybe lack of sleep and the paucity of time with loved ones are holding your health back and stoking disconnection syndrome. Maybe you're a workaholic who hasn't left the building and gone on a nature-filled walk in years. Or you're tethered to your digital devices and know you could use a break from social media. Certain lessons in this book are going to speak to you. And we will give you plenty of strategies for tailoring the lessons to your own life — the tools, as it were, to switch gears.

SWITCHING GEARS

<u>David</u>: I learned many life lessons during my first year of neurosurgery training. It was the mid-1980s, and the demands placed upon us were immense. We residents would work thirty-six hours, then have twelve hours off, often for several weeks at a time. To say that I was not getting enough restorative sleep is an understatement. This lack of sleep, coupled with the stress of work, was unquestionably destabilizing my health. And with little time to

focus on consuming high-quality food, I soon became sick. During that year, the first health issue I experienced was the development of esophagitis, an inflammatory disease of the esophagus that makes swallowing—even drinking water—incredibly painful. Next came dysentery, a severe illness characterized by high fever and diarrhea. In my case, the degree of dehydration I experienced was so severe that I remained on intravenous fluids for several days. As I began to recover, I contracted chicken pox.

At that point, I began considering a career change. Soon thereafter, while having dinner one night at my parents' home, another illness descended on me. While we were having our meal, I grew increasingly uncomfortable and shortly thereafter developed incredible pain—specifically, in my testicles. This pain far exceeded anything I had ever experienced, including while playing contact sports, so my parents and I decided that I should go to an emergency room. It was there that I was diagnosed with mumps, a disease that could have made me sterile.

Looking back, I know that without question, my health was severely jeopardized by lack of sleep, chronic stress, poor dietary choices, and an almost total absence of exposure to nature. Although I didn't undergo any blood testing to evaluate the level of inflammation in my body, I have no doubt that my markers would have been extremely high. Fortunately, the change I needed to make was clear. I decided to switch from neurosurgery to neurology, a specialty in which I could have better control of my time (and life). I truly believe that that simple decision saved me. And while so many maladaptive lifestyle events have conspired to bring me down, I've learned over the years that not every lifestyle factor has to be compromised in order for a person to manifest illness. A bad diet, not enough restorative sleep, or unrelenting stress, individually, can be devastating.

Even on days when we're dealing with serious challenges or setbacks, or when we experience a disappointment or loss, we can still live with an undercurrent of optimism and contentment. Happiness and frustration are not mutually exclusive. But we cannot feel authentically joyful while being impetuous, lonely, narcissistic, indifferent, and dispassionate. Those descriptors cannot coexist. They keep us disconnected, and they keep us sick.

The health issues of the modern world are more than the list of individual conditions in a textbook. True health is a vibrant state of mental and physical well-being that transcends any specific diagnosis. This place of wellness is found through deep connection to ourselves, to others, and to the living space that we share with all humans. In order to get there, we need to take a close look at the central player: the brain.

CHAPTER 2

Mind Blowing

The Incredible History of Your Brain

*Very little is needed to make a happy life; it is all within
yourself, in your way of thinking.*

—Marcus Aurelius

In a single second, our brains fire off a dazzling
number of signals, propelling essential information
through our neurons at up to 268 miles per hour.
Neurons—basic cells of the nervous system that send
and receive communications through chemical and
electrical impulses—fire at a staggering rate relative to
our slow-beating heart. It's remarkable, really, when we
pause to appreciate the human brain, an encapsu-
lated three-pound organ that contains more connections than there are stars in the known galaxy. It creates
our entire experience of life, constantly helping us
make sense of an unbelievably complicated and ever-
changing world and making decisions for us before we

are even aware of them. Our exquisite brains have allowed us to thrive on this planet in the face of countless challenges, including real threats to our survival.

In modernized countries, we've removed most of the barriers to basic needs and potentially life-threatening dangers. This has theoretically given us the opportunity to focus on developing purpose, joy, and enduring health. But as we learned in the previous chapter, we face epidemics of loneliness, depression, anxiety, addiction, and chronic, preventable disease. This sad state of affairs has arisen because the brain's long-established processes that allowed for our survival over the course of millions of years have been hijacked by aspects of contemporary life. This mental hijacking keeps us constantly craving instant gratification and in a perpetual and unnecessary state of stress, fear, and discontent. As we discussed in chapter 1, we are calling this disconnection syndrome. We're going to show you how this happens at the level of your brain's wiring and start to teach you solutions for taking back control so you can live a more fulfilling, happy, and engaged life.

Without a doubt, your day-to-day existence is defined by the experiences and interactions that fill your waking hours. All these moments require processing before you can make sense of them. The brain's one-hundred-billion-plus neurons are able to accomplish this by using neurotransmitters—chemical signaling molecules that allow for the transfer of messages across the brain. These messages also are modified by hormones, another set of chemical messengers that affect the brain and the rest of the body. Collectively, neurotransmitters and hormones work together, driving feelings of joy, anger, bliss, hunger, lust, and desire. These molecules are absolutely influenced by your food, sleep, physical movement, and interactions with your environment and other people. They are also affected by your levels of stress, feelings of gratitude, and sense of empathy and compassion for others. When any signaling pathway—whether in the brain or elsewhere in the body—is defective or somehow out of balance, you can suffer consequences to your health and even your behavior. Let's describe this biology, focusing squarely on the main command center: the brain.

WHAT FIRES TOGETHER WIRES TOGETHER

The brain is an electrical marvel. Each moment, electrical signals zip down your neurons to convey information between your brain cells. When each signal reaches the end of the neuron, a chemical messenger called a neurotransmitter is released into the tiny gap, called a synapse, that links neurons. These gaps are complex zones of constant communication between neurons, and the strength of this communication determines how tightly neurons are linked. Examples of common neurotransmitters that you'll be reading about include dopamine, serotonin, adrenaline, noradrenaline, and endorphins.

Each neuron can form thousands of links to neighboring brain cells, giving a typical human brain trillions of synapses. Neurotransmitters are received in neighboring cells by dendrites, which convert the neurotransmitters back into electrical signals, and the message moves on. This complex wiring allows neurons to communicate with one another and generate biological wonders such as thought, sensation, and movement.

One of the most revelatory discoveries of our lifetimes has been that the brain is plastic, meaning it can reorganize itself by forming new neural connections throughout a person's life. It's pliable, impressionable, *moldable*. This means you can change the wiring of your brain right now. As it is said in neurology circles, neurons that fire together wire together: when one brain cell sends signals to another, the connection between the two gets stronger. The more signals sent between them, the more robust the connection becomes. Every time you experience something new, your brain slightly rewires to accommodate that new experience. And the more you engage in a particular activity, the more indelible and *influential* the connections needed to perform that activity become. In simplest terms, **the more you do something, the more you do something.** This is true whether that something is good or bad for you.

In fact, the way you choose to use your brain helps determine how your brain is organized overall. As you learn and experience the world, the links among your neurons are modified. New connections are created while unused connections die off. This is how we build a more efficient brain. It constantly and dynamically shapes and reshapes itself—both structurally and functionally—in response to experiences, learning, and even injury. Our good friend Dr. Michael Merzenich, a neuroscientist and pioneer in brain plasticity research, describes it perfectly in Sharon Begley's *Train Your Mind, Change Your Brain*: "Experience coupled with attention leads to physical changes in the structure and future functioning of the nervous system. This leaves us with a clear physiological fact... moment by moment we choose and sculpt how our ever-changing minds will work. We choose who we will be in the next moment in a very real sense, and these choices are left embossed in physical form in our material selves."[1]

Dr. Merzenich's description of plasticity is a key point, because it means that neuroplasticity—the ability of the brain to form and organize synaptic connections—can either work for or against us. That is, if we choose to engage in activities that constantly bombard us with negativity or provoke a sense of fear, our brains will be rewired to respond to this negativity and fear-driven state. In the cogent words of His Holiness the 14th Dalai Lama, "The brain we develop reflects the life we lead."

If you're wondering just how the brain enhances and protects its connections, it's largely through the help of a protein called brain-derived neurotrophic factor, or BDNF. In the brain, BDNF is active at the synaptic connections. Much of what science knows about this protein comes from studying people who suffer from a lack of it. For example, studies have demonstrated decreased levels of BDNF in Alzheimer's disease patients.[2] This is an illness that world-renowned neurodegenerative disease expert Dr. Dale Bredesen has indicated is characterized primarily by the loss of connections (synapses) between brain cells.[3] And we'll be connecting the dots so you can see how disconnection syndrome may be a factor in the development of diseases like Alzheimer's. Indeed, preventing cognitive decline is very much in line with the central premise of this book—preserving and amplifying purpose, joy, and health across one's life span. Optimizing brain health to preserve our thinking and intellect is critical: it's the goal of the Brain Wash program.

In light of this, it should be no surprise that scientists are looking for ways to increase BDNF in the brain. It turns out that our lifestyle choices are highly influential in this regard. You can harness this amazing bit of information to form new connections in your brain, targeting critical areas such as the prefrontal cortex to help you make good, conscious decisions based on what you've learned from past experience and what you can expect from potential future consequences. The Brain

Wash program will include strategies to increase your BDNF so you can change your brain.

OUR THREE BRAINS

In addition to being an electrical marvel, the brain is also an evolutionary wonder. You can think of yourself as having three separate brains, each reflecting a different stage in human evolution.[4] The current scientifically accepted model of brain activity is more complex, but the simplicity of the three-brain model is helpful for the purposes of our discussion.

Our Original Brain

Our first and oldest brain dates back to the time of prehistoric reptiles (go ahead, think dinosaurs). We continue to share this part of the brain with modern reptiles and birds. In humans, this part of the brain is housed in the brainstem. Not surprisingly, it governs very basic but vital functions and receives direct input from the entire body. For example, the brainstem is involved in the regulation of our heartbeat, breathing, blood pressure, circulation, digestion, and the famous fight-or-flight response. What stands out about this part of the brain is that it's strictly instinctual and automatic. It is critical to our survival but doesn't require us to think or feel in order to work.

Our Limbic Brain

It wasn't until we evolved into mammals that the next level of brain development occurred. This would become the limbic brain, which sits on top of the brainstem and receives input from the old reptilian brain below.

The limbic brain generates emotions based on sensory input. Like those of the brainstem, the limbic brain's responses are automatic and frequently reflexive—without conscious analysis, reflection, or interpretation. These responses developed out of a need for preservation and survival. Within the limbic brain we find the physical and emotional basis for primal experiences such as hunger, pain, sleepiness, anger, fear, and pleasure.

One thing that makes the limbic brain so significant is that it's associated with the release of the neurotransmitter dopamine and the brain's natural opiates, called endorphins. Much more information on these important chemical messengers is coming in the next chapter, but suffice it to say that one of the many functions of dopamine is that it strongly influences our "reward circuits" and behaviors, including our habits and, yes, addictions. Reward circuits are pathways in the brain that govern our responses to rewards such as food, sex, and social interactions. As we'll soon see, dopamine plays a central role in our incessant need for instant gratification and in the development of addiction. Pleasure-inducing chemicals like the feel-good endorphins, which act on the body's opiate receptors, are also involved. When we experience something that initiates the reward circuit, these brain chemicals influence the brain and body to continue seeking out whatever stimuli are generating the pleasurable sensation.

The limbic system is not a single structure. Scientists have debated the specific components of the limbic system, but most descriptions include the amygdala, hippocampus, thalamus, hypothalamus, and cingulate gyrus. All these components work together to control some of the brain's most important processes. You don't need to understand all this anatomy or even how these structures collaborate in scientific detail. We'll be simplifying what you need to know for the purposes of our discussion, and we'll be homing in on the area of the limbic brain that has received a substantial amount of attention: the *amygdala*.

The amygdala has been the subject of much study for several decades. When scientists intentionally damage the amygdala in research animals, they find the animals lose their aggressive behavior and their ability to react normally to fear. They become fearless. Although such studies in monkeys date back decades, only recently have we documented similar findings in humans. In 2010, an unusual human case allowed scientists to confirm that a missing amygdala has behavioral consequences.[5] A forty-four-year-old woman, code-named patient SM to protect her privacy, suffered a rare condition that led to an absence of brain tissue in the place where her amygdala would normally reside. Not only did she lack fear of creatures such as snakes and spiders, she would also put her life at risk without any apparent concern. In one instance, she walked through a park alone at night and was attacked by a man with a knife. The following day, she again walked through the same park. World-famous climber Alex Honnold, whose Academy Award–winning documentary, *Free Solo*, chronicles his climb up Yosemite National Park's Half Dome alone without a rope, owes some of his fearlessness to the way in which his brain fires. Turns out his amygdala doesn't activate normally.[6] It remains relatively quiet during his sensation-seeking adventures, during which death is a real possibility. A normally functioning amygdala might well keep him away from those death-defying ledges.

The amygdala is the control center of the threat-response and threat-interpretation system. It modulates our memories of threatening events, real or perceived. To be clear, the limbic system's hippocampus is the main memory center, but the nearby amygdala participates: these brain structures are activated following an emotional event and "talk" with each other in the process of memory consolidation. Memories in general, whether they elicit strong emotions or not, also involve the prefrontal cortex. Interactions between the hippocampus and prefrontal cortex support the assimilation of new memories into preexisting networks of knowledge, ultimately providing the foundation of memory consolidation — and later retrieval.

But the amygdala helps record real or perceived threats as well as other emotion-filled experiences so that we can recognize similar events in the future. As an example, think of a time when you hit the car brakes as soon as your eyes detected a large object on the road. In cases like this, we rely on an instantaneous, automatic response that doesn't require conscious decision making. This type of response is part of our survival instinct.

DAVID'S AMYGDALA

Several years ago I learned an important life lesson. My wife and I had just about finished shopping at Costco. We were in line with our cart and were almost ready to check out. My wife suddenly realized that there was one last item that she had forgotten, so she went to retrieve it while I waited in line. When she returned, the fact that she had left the line must have violated some rule in the mind of the man who was waiting behind us, despite the fact that the cashier was still not ready for us. He proceeded to look at me and spew negative comments. I ignored him.

Then he turned his aggression away from me and directed it to my wife. Accosting her the way he did instantly disconnected my brain from rationality and thoughtful response. I was in full attack mode when I approached him, and by the grace of God, he must've sensed it. He immediately raised his palms and backed off. Fortunately, I was able to regain control, and the situation was defused. I had a lot to think about on the drive home that day.

With its powerful relationship to emotion and fear, one might expect that abnormal functioning of the amygdala—resulting from developmental problems, neurotransmitter imbalance, or structural damage— might be linked to conditions such as depression, PTSD, phobias, anxiety, and impulsivity, and that is in fact the case. But here's the important lesson: **the circuit in the amygdala can be hacked or altered** even in an otherwise healthy brain. **And when it's tinkered with, big problems ensue.** Anxiety, for example, is an amygdala-based response to something that is only *perceived* as being dangerous because of a previous experience. Panic attacks can occur when the amygdala is sending danger signals even though in reality no such danger exists. And the amygdala doesn't just play a role in mental health issues. We're going to show you how too much activation of this part of your brain can interfere with your ability to make good decisions and control your emotions. Most important, we're going to show you how to tame your amygdala so you can reclaim your life.

The amygdala is a central influencer of emotion, impulsivity, and reward. An overactive amygdala is an essential part of the story that has led us to our current societal predicament. But the brain is not a collection of siloed parts and functions. The amygdala drives our response to fear-inducing events and our ability to remember these events, but it works in concert with other areas of the brain, including the prefrontal cortex.

Our Third Brain

In the most recent, third stage of evolution, mammals developed a new part of the brain on top of the limbic brain—the cerebral cortex. When you picture a human brain, you likely see lots of folds and creases. That's the cerebral cortex you're looking at. The more folds, the greater the surface area of the brain and the more advanced its capabilities. It is this part of the brain that gives us high-reasoning abilities—the ability to think analytically and logically, problem solve, plan for the future, and think abstractly. This most highly evolved part of the brain regulates and attempts to control impulses of the older, more primitive brain. This is called top-down brain functioning.

The emergence of our "new" third brain provided us with a much-needed counterbalance to the limbic brain, giving us a spectacular new set of survival skills. The cerebral cortex is, as its name implies, the cerebral part of us — it's reflective, contemplative, and methodical. The prefrontal cortex is a key part of the cerebral cortex. Its complexity is a unique attribute of humans. It takes up about 10 percent of the total volume of the brain, and, as we noted previously, it occupies nearly one-third of the entire neocortex. Like a CEO who directs the many employees and operations under his or her watch, the prefrontal cortex attempts to find the best possible response to incoming information. It allows us to make a plan that weighs alternatives instead of immediately reacting to circumstances. This process defines executive function and is the exact opposite of the functions carried out by the reactive amygdala.

The amygdala and prefrontal cortex are in constant communication. The connection between these two areas influences our behavior as well as our ability to regulate impulsivity and emotion. When the balance of activity becomes too one-sided and the amygdala's primal responses dominate unchecked, trouble looms. For example, scientists have found that a weak connection between the amygdala and the prefrontal cortex is linked to anxiety.[7] Without the supervision of the prefrontal cortex, there's no adult in the room. The emotionally immature child can run amok, lacking rules, discipline, and boundaries.

Research is showing that the relationship between the amygdala and the prefrontal cortex is actively being sabotaged by the chronic stress and lack of adequate

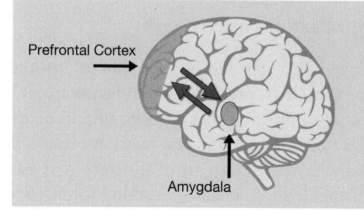

sleep that are so characteristic of modern life.[8] Unhealthful digital exposure, nature deprivation, and poor diet only add to the problem. This is threatening not just us as individuals but also the health of the entire planet. As we'll soon see, people with relatively inactive prefrontal cortices may be less concerned about the planet's health than others are. They are, simply put, selfish in every sense of the word—from the way they treat others to the way they treat the environment. When we are able to actively use our prefrontal cortices in decision making, we can become more compassionate and empathic individuals. This is significant and offers the opportunity for a paradigm shift.

> The shift away from the prefrontal cortex represents the gravest existential threat for human survival.

The Curious Case of Phineas Gage

Phineas Gage (1823–60) has become a fixture in the curricula of neurology, psychology, and neuroscience.[9] His story is so compelling that it's been told in many lay circles as well. And though you may have heard of him, we want to tell you a part of his story that has rarely been highlighted. It has everything to do with our subject matter and the power of neuroplasticity. First, a quick refresher on the life of Mr. Gage.

Mr. Gage was a railroad construction worker. While blasting rock for one of his jobs, he suffered a terrible accident in which a large iron rod was driven completely through his head. The rod entered just below his left cheekbone and exited on the left side of the top of his skull. Thirty minutes after the event, a physician, Edward Williams, saw him. Dr. Williams wrote the following about his encounter with Mr. Gage:[10]

> When I drove up, he said, "Doctor, here is business enough for you." I first noticed the wound upon the head before I alighted from my carriage, the pulsations of the brain being very distinct... the top of the head appeared somewhat like an inverted funnel... the whole wound appeared as if some wedge-shaped body had passed from below upward. Mr. Gage, during the time I was examining this wound, was relating the manner in which he was injured to the bystanders....

About this time, Mr. G. got up and vomited... the effort of vomiting pressed out about half a tea-cupfull of the brain [through the exit hole at the top of the skull], which fell upon the floor.

Incredibly, even though this happened in the mid-1800s, Mr. Gage survived his injury and lived for almost thirteen more years. What became so instructive and has remained enlightening was how this event affected the understanding of brain function, especially as it relates to personality. Mr. Gage's personality suffered a temporary blow following the accident, which caused serious trauma to his prefrontal cortex. As documented, he had been an upstanding, emotionally stable individual prior to the injury, but immediately thereafter he was noted to be intractable, impatient, vulgar, and lacking empathy. According to Dr. John Martyn Harlow, the physician who ultimately took care of Mr. Gage after his injury:[11]

The equilibrium or balance, so to speak, between his intellectual faculties and animal propensities, seems to have been destroyed. He is fitful, irreverent, indulging at times in the grossest profanity (which was not previously his custom), manifesting but little deference for his fellows, impatient of restraint or advice when it conflicts with his desires, at times pertinaciously obstinate, yet capricious and vacillating, devising many plans of future operations, which are no sooner arranged than they are abandoned in turn for others appearing more feasible. A child in his intellectual capacity and manifestations, he has the animal passions of a strong man. Previous to his injury, although untrained in the schools, he possessed a well-balanced mind, and was looked upon by those who knew him as a shrewd, smart business man, very energetic and persistent in executing all his plans of operation. In this regard his mind was radically changed, so decidedly that his friends and acquaintances said he was "no longer Gage."

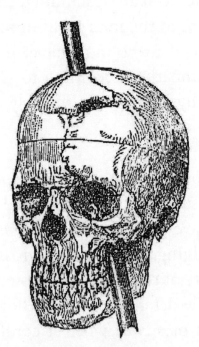

"Recovery from the Passage of an Iron Bar through the Head."

This story is often used to illustrate the unique functional properties of the amygdala and the prefrontal cortex. Mr. Gage went from being an even-tempered gentleman to an irreverent, impetuous human being because of the breakdown of his prefrontal cortex upon injury. His amygdala was able to fire unchecked, without the benefit of calming, rational input from the prefrontal cortex.

But there's part of the story that is less well known but extremely illuminating and further instructive. After the injury, Mr. Gage spent many years working as a stagecoach driver in Chile. He was described in later life as having regained some of his social graces. This clearly shows that the brain can heal and change in the right environment—it is a testament to the power of neuroplasticity. Mr. Gage was seemingly able to reestablish connection to his prefrontal cortex despite traumatic injury. He didn't die in a fit of rage or succumb to an impulsive leap off a bridge. He died following a series of seizures that was likely part of the injury's long-term effects. Today the rod that went through his head is on display at the Harvard Medical School's Warren Anatomical Museum.

The Phineas Gage story is a dramatic one, but from this extraordinary tale we can draw parallels to modern life. Just as Mr. Gage became disconnected from his prefrontal cortex through a physical wound, we, too, become disconnected from the prefrontal cortex in ways that we'll explore in detail. The good news is that we can, like Mr. Gage, reconnect by rewiring, regaining, retraining, and restrengthening that connection thanks to neuroplasticity. We can "wash out" the wounds and heal.

The observations in the Phineas Gage case were made without the benefit of modern technology, but they nevertheless clued us in to a totally new view of the brain. Today we have access to many advanced tools for studying the brain. A whole new field of research is in fact emerging to study—and perhaps capitalize on—the power of the prefrontal cortex. Fascinating new research shows that when people have noninvasive, low-energy electrical currents pulsed through their heads targeting specific areas of the brain (technically called transcranial direct current stimulation, or tDCS), the brain's functionality changes almost instantly and self-regulation improves (note: this form of therapy uses low levels of electrical current and is completely different from electroconvulsive therapy, or ECT). In a 2019 study conducted by a global team of researchers from the University of Oxford, Harvard Medical School, and the University of California at Berkeley and published in the *Journal of the American Medical Association,* a group of women suffering from anxiety underwent a single session of electrical stimulation of their prefrontal cortices.[12] As a result, their amygdalas' fear signaling decreased while their attention control increased. Attention control is a fancy way of saying "ability to concentrate and choose what to pay attention to versus ignore."

This study showed that enhancing the prefrontal cortex's activity ultimately helps manage responses to perceived threats. Put simply, the world becomes less scary, and we are less reactive—especially when being reactive is not warranted. In a 2019 review of brain-stimulation studies, the scientists state: "Self-regulation...enable[s] individuals to guide their thoughts, feelings, and behaviors in a purposeful manner. Self-regulation is crucial for goal-directed behavior and has been related to many consequential outcomes in life including physical and mental health, psychological well-being, ethical decision making, and strong interpersonal relationships...[S]timulating the prefrontal cortex promotes successful self-regulation by altering the balance in activity between the prefrontal cortex and subcortical regions involved in emotion and reward processing [a.k.a., the amygdala and reward systems]."[13]

This type of research could have remarkable clinical applications. People with anxiety disorders, for example, could potentially use this noninvasive, drug-free approach to not only manage their conditions but also improve the parts of their brains that render them better able to focus, make good decisions, and generally see the world as a kinder place. At the moment, this kind of electrical stimulation is still being evaluated for efficacy and safety. The important message, however, is that activation of the prefrontal cortex is a powerful force for improving your life. And bringing that about is likely something each of us can control.

Early Life Stress

Although we wouldn't want to intentionally damage the amygdala–prefrontal cortex connection in humans, we have gained important insights from victims of early life stress. In a 2018 study, researchers from a group of institutions including the University of Pennsylvania and the Massachusetts Institute of Technology explored the ways in which childhood adversity—defined as the death of a family member, parental conflict, or a serious accident— might affect the connection between the amygdala and the prefrontal cortex and the ways in which damage to this connection might relate to issues such as aggressive behavior and attention problems.[14] Stressful situations in childhood are a clear risk factor for mental health disorders, and researchers wanted to determine if a damaged amygdala–prefrontal cortex connection could explain this risk. In their study, the researchers performed MRI scans on seventy-nine children between the ages of four and seven, using questionnaires to assess the presence of stressful life events, aggressive behavior, attention problems, anxiety, and depression. The results of the study were telling. First, they demonstrated that exposure to stressful life events was significantly correlated with a weak connection between the amygdala and the prefrontal cortex. In addition, such stress exposure was strongly correlated with increased levels of aggressive behavior and attention problems and "symptoms of poorer mental health." In an important observation, the researchers pointed out that their findings were similar to those seen in older children and adolescents. They concluded: "Our results suggest that abnormal amygdala functional connectivity in young children could be a potential marker of latent risk for poor emotion regulation capacity, and may manifest as clinically relevant symptoms later in life."[15]

The effects of chronic stress on the prefrontal cortex are powerful, and they don't just stem from childhood trauma. Other kinds of stressors can weaken the connection to the prefrontal cortex and even damage the prefrontal cortex itself, allowing the amygdala to function unchecked.

Understanding the story of the prefrontal cortex and the amygdala is key as we move ahead to untangle the question of how modern influences modify our health and happiness. In the chapters to come, we'll show you how to use this information to activate your prefrontal cortex and tame the amygdala. Before we do this, though, we need to explain how disconnection syndrome affects not only our brain's connectivity but also its underlying chemical messaging and reward system. Let's go there next.

CHAPTER 3

The Brain's Highs and Lows

The Route to Reward

Do not bite at the bait of pleasure till you know there is no hook beneath it.

—THOMAS JEFFERSON

IF YOU COULD TIME-TRAVEL BACK twelve thousand years, before the advent of agriculture, and ask humans about the last time they felt the pleasures of a natural high, you might hear about sex or about a great hunt and kill followed by a celebratory feast with friends around a fire.

Although they didn't know its name at the time, your ancestors would be telling you about the activation of a mechanism in the body aptly called the reward pathway. Indeed, rewards lead to pleasure. They are experienced in response to discrete stimuli, providing enjoyment and arousal. This part of our biology is essential to our evolutionary development. Its function—to promote life-sustaining activities such as finding food and water, engaging in sex for reproduction, and taking care of our newborn babies—has been key to ensuring the survival of *Homo sapiens* across the millennia. And leading scientific research has now provided a better understanding of the actual hardwiring of this long-established brain system. Unfortunately, this also means that people have become extremely adept at exploiting it.

Now that you've gotten a sense of your brain's old and new biology, let's go deeper into its chemistry to understand how you can become addicted to things that keep you from vibrant well-being.

THE POWER OF PLEASURE

Your brain responds to any pleasurable experience in a uniform, deliberate way. It follows a script that was written into the body's operating system eons ago. The neurotransmitter dopamine gets released from the ventral tegmental area, or VTA, a small clump of neurons that sits midbrain. From there, dopamine zooms to many different parts of the brain. It goes to the amygdala and hippocampus, the two structures heavily involved in emotions and memory formation. But most important for the purposes of our discussion, it travels to another important structure in the reward circuitry called the nucleus accumbens, which is a collection of neurons directly involved with the experience of pleasure. And it reaches the prefrontal cortex, which, as you know, helps focus attention and planning. When you experience a stimulus that triggers the reward circuit, dopamine is released, leading to a cascade of chemical messaging that essentially tells the body to follow through on obtaining the reward and to remember to do it again. This reward system is complicated, but we're going to try our best to keep it simple.

Dopamine is a critical piece of the reward system. However, despite what you might have heard, the scientific consensus is that dopamine is not responsible for creating the feeling of pleasure. Instead, elevated dopamine seems to generate a strong sense of wanting or craving. That said, some rewards do activate endogenous opioid peptides (EOPs), which, like the drug morphine, bring about a sensation of pleasure. These are the brain's natural opiates. Here's the important thing about the reward circuit: the pathway can easily be overactivated by modern-day activities such as gambling and even shopping. When this happens, the dopamine system is adversely altered and knocked off balance, leading to cravings and eventually resulting in addictive behaviors. Of course, different stimuli activate this circuitry in different ways and to varying degrees. For example, drugs such as heroin and cocaine lead to greater dependency than others because they activate the reward circuit more intensely.

The hippocampus, amygdala, prefrontal cortex, and nucleus accumbens all have receptors for dopamine. As you might guess, dopamine affects each of these parts of the brain differently. Though scientists are piecing together exactly how it works, here's one simplified way of looking at what's probably taking place in your brain: your amygdala interprets an experience as positive, and your hippocampus responds by committing the experience to memory so it can be repeated. Meanwhile, your nucleus accumbens lights up with activity as dopamine levels rise, and it urges you to keep doing what you're doing. To give one example, say you eat a big spoonful of ice cream. It's delicious beyond measure. Your amygdala notes that it makes you feel good while your hippocampus registers what you did to obtain that ice cream so you remember how to get it again, and your nucleus accumbens encourages you to take another bite. Meanwhile, your prefrontal cortex helps you stay focused on finishing the ice cream. The reward circuitry keeps spinning.

The Law of Diminishing Returns

As the reward pathway remains activated and dopamine keeps surging, eventually there's a law of diminishing returns to contend with. This is why some drugs can be so problematic. The most addictive drugs, for example, cause brain cells to massively increase the release of dopamine, along with other pleasure-inducing brain chemicals. The brain compensates for this by lowering the production of dopamine and decreasing the number of available receptors for it to bind to. This means that the next time the drug is used, the effect won't be as strong—the user has built up a *tolerance* to it. Unfortunately, this also causes the user to increase his or her drug use in order to get that same high. As the brain continues to adapt to these drugs, the regions of the brain responsible for judgment and memory are also changed. This hardwiring makes drug-seeking behavior a habit, setting the stage for addiction.

But the drugs of today are not just classic addictive substances such as opioids and alcohol. Anything that repeatedly overactivates this powerful circuitry will change the brain and have major consequences. As we know, craving-related behavior is not always beneficial. When we find ourselves pleasure seeking 24-7, chasing instant gratification and pushing those chemical buttons, we reinforce neural pathways that keep us constantly craving and silence the prefrontal cortex by weakening its ability to exert control over the lower, limbic brain. And this manifests itself, among other ways, as internet surfing, smartphone scrolling, one-click shopping, gobbling up high-calorie foods, and checking posts on social media.

Striking a Balance

The brain is constantly striving to keep your various neurochemical systems in balance, something it does through ongoing neurobiological and synaptic shifts that alter the levels of neurotransmitters in the brain. There's a rhythm of "upregulation" and "downregulation." For example, during the night, when you need to sleep, the inhibitory neurotransmitter GABA (gamma-aminobutyric acid) blocks the activity of neurotransmitters that are active during wakefulness. During the day, when you need to be alert, think, and react, the brain rebalances itself so these other neurotransmitters are removed from sleep-based inhibitory control.

It is when these various systems become imbalanced or somehow artificially manipulated that we begin to go down a dangerous path. When one system cannot speak to another—when the wiring is askew—cognitive function, including the way we think, act, feel, and make decisions, worsens. We'll show you plenty of examples of this cause and effect. For now, let's turn to the stress response system, which has everything to do with dopamine-driven behaviors, especially as they relate to feeling "low" or anxious.

The Doldrums of Our Survival Instinct

A lot of us are living in a perpetual state of anxiety and disquietude. This isn't surprising. As we'll soon see, being sleep-deprived and surrounded by a constant flow of negative news not only puts us into a primal "survival mode" but also creates profound downstream effects on our brain's wiring and resulting behaviors. Here's the gist.

When we experience stress or feel fearful, our bodies respond by releasing a variety of chemicals. At center stage is the hormone cortisol. Cortisol triggers many biological actions, affecting our blood sugar and influencing immune function. The classic fight-or-flight reaction sets in when adrenaline and noradrenaline (a.k.a. norepinephrine) flood the system, raising heart rate and blood pressure and changing the flow of blood throughout the body. This primes us to deal with the stressor. Like the reward pathway, the stress-response pathway is one of the most established and hardwired processes of our evolution.

So what happens to the brain's circuitry when we're exposed to stress? The amygdala activates stress pathways, which in turn impair prefrontal cortex regulation and strengthen amygdala function. This generates a vicious cycle in which high levels of stress keep the amygdala in the driver's seat. Our brain's response patterns switch from slow, thoughtful prefrontal cortex control to the reflexive and rapid emotional responses of the amygdala and related limbic structures. This explains why we become impulsive, irrational, and generally worse decision makers when we are stressed.

What is most critical to understand is that when we

are chronically stressed, we're basically giving the reins of our lives to the amygdala, allowing it to influence an increasing number of our decisions. Stress is like fuel for the amygdala and poison for the prefrontal cortex. In animal studies, chronic stress leads to changes in the physical structure of the prefrontal cortex, rendering it increasingly unable to suppress the impulsive amygdala.[1] Meanwhile, it also promotes new neuron growth in the amygdala.[2] And what happens as the amygdala gets stronger? We have trouble making wise, well-thought-out decisions, creating more long-term stress and perpetuating the problem. This is how disconnection syndrome takes hold. As described in an eye-opening paper in *Nature Neuroscience,* "This flip from reflective to reflexive brain state may have survival value when we are in danger, but it can be ruinous for life in the Information Age, when we need higher cognitive abilities to thrive."[3]

As this stress-induced remodeling of the brain is allowed to continue, we pursue short-term quick fixes driven strongly by the hunt for pleasure and the avoidance of pain.

What's most interesting about this whole cascade is that stress greatly increases dopamine release.[4] As we've mentioned, too much dopamine over time can alter and damage the dopamine system, pushing us toward unhealthful, craving-fueled behavior. For example, we might binge on high-carb foods as a way to reestablish balance in the dopamine system. Living in a chronic state of heightened amygdala-based reactions makes us vulnerable to developing patterns, habits, and routines that attempt to manage these reactions, and this leaves us feeling out of control and overwhelmed.

Now let's take a close look at some of the behaviors that create and reinforce disconnection syndrome. We will be going into much greater depth in subsequent chapters, but a preview will help you grasp what's really going on in your brain.

A DAY IN A DISCONNECTED LIFE

The average American wakes up to a sleep deficit. In addition to the many well-established health consequences of poor or insufficient sleep (more on this later), a sleep deficit increases production of the hormone cortisol. Cortisol, as we just mentioned, is a stress hormone and a key component of the fight-or-flight response. High morning cortisol levels are shown to be associated with depressive symptoms as well as a general feeling of stress. At the microscopic level, cortisol influences glucose and fat metabolism and plays a role in the functioning of our immune systems. What's more, high cortisol levels are found in a variety of disease processes and are commonly associated with greater overall metabolic stress on the body. Most relevant to our discussion, and as we described above, stress empowers the amygdala while directly threatening the prefrontal cortex.

What do we do once we wake up? Fully 79 percent of adults reach for their smartphones in the first fifteen minutes after waking up.[5] That number climbs to 89 percent among people between the ages of eighteen and twenty-four.[6] Right away, we satisfy the craving to check our phones—a result of the dopamine surge. How many people liked our last Instagram post? Who texted us? What calls did we miss? How many emails have come in since last night? We are conditioned to expect immediate gratification.

Survey data indicate that for the 34 percent of Americans who eat breakfast every day, the most common choice is cold cereal. Data also indicate that a third of us feel rushed when we eat.[7] Almost all cereal, especially cereal designed for children, has had sugar added to it. This is *cereal* we're talking about, a product often touted as healthful. Many people instead reach for doughnuts, muffins, or other highly processed breakfast desserts to start their days. If you drink coffee, that's fine, but if you're drinking mocha lattes and ice-blended coffee drinks, you might as well be having a sugary milk shake. Large datasets indicate that these types of high-glycemic-index foods—foods that increase blood sugar quickly—may themselves contribute to depression.[8] They do so through inflammation pathways.

As we will later learn, inflammation antagonizes the

actions of the important neurotransmitter serotonin. It's vital to note that it also threatens our ability to employ the prefrontal cortex. Case in point: in a 2018 study conducted at Emory University, researchers used functional MRI on patients suffering from depression. Inflammation was found to be associated with a significant reduction in the strength of the connection between the amygdala and the prefrontal cortex.[9] In addition, inflammation appears to increase the amygdala's response to threatening images.[10] Such findings become all the more meaningful when we consider the multitude of ways inflammation is amped up in our bodies, including poor choices in food, sleep deprivation, an inactive lifestyle, and lack of exposure to nature, to name a few. Anything that enhances inflammation may threaten our ability to use our prefrontal cortices, leaving the amygdala to its own devices. This means we lose the benefit of the prefrontal cortex in helping dial down our impulsive behavior.

The science connecting inflammation and behavioral lapses such as poor decision making and impulsivity is hot off the presses of our medical journals. We know that chronic inflammation affects the entire body and is strongly tied to diseases such as depression and dementia. It's not surprising that inflammation would also be linked to the day-to-day function of our decision-making and advanced thinking processes. Which makes anything that foments inflammation and disrupts or co-opts our prefrontal cortices all the more suspect.

Our ancestors probably didn't have to deal with chronic inflammation, at least not as we do today. As such, our bodies didn't evolve to deal effectively with exposure to long-term inflammation. How can we prevent chronic inflammation? One good place to start is our food choices.

> Inflammation's ripple effects in the brain may ultimately translate to our having less control over our actions and emotions.

Food Is Behavioral Information

The idea that **what we eat threatens our ability to access the prefrontal cortex** should be a game changer in itself. It means quite literally that our diets can put us at risk for becoming more self-centered and less empathic. More hedonistic and less restrained. Food is, in a real sense, dictating our behaviors! Diets high in refined carbohydrates are also linked to myriad other health issues, including increased risk of stroke, heart disease, and diabetes. We're trying to fuel ourselves for success, but we're really just powering disease.

We should note that our food cravings — especially

for sweet, sugary foods—have their roots in our ancestry. Our desire for sugar is hardwired because it represents a potent survival mechanism. It proved extremely helpful for our hunter-gatherer forebears to actively seek out the proverbial fig tree. Sugar, or something sweet, was an indication that fruit was ripe. This meant that our ancestors would eat fruit at the peak of its nutritional value. Typically, this would occur in the late summer and fall, and the sugar would help our ancestors produce and store body fat. This fat provided an energy reservoir during the caloric scarcity of winter, creating an important survival advantage. Sweetness also has another important characteristic: it means "safe." There are virtually no poisonous sweet fruits, so sweetness *was* an important quality to seek out.

Sweetness dramatically activates the brain's dopamine reward pathway, as has been demonstrated using sophisticated brain-imaging technology.[11] And, as you know now, the more this pathway is rewarded, the more it needs to be stimulated. Why do you think you still want a sugar-rich dessert even after you've eaten a full meal? How is it you can barely finish what's on your dinner plate but have no problem polishing off that large piece of chocolate cake afterward? To make matters worse, overstimulation of the reward system alters dopamine signaling, leading to addictive symptoms. Along with changes in the dopamine receptors, this process seems to weaken the prefrontal cortex, rendering it less able to control impulsive urges and addictive tendencies.[12] To summarize, sugar (and the simple carbohydrates that your body rapidly converts into sugar) powerfully hacks into your reward pathway, altering your neurochemistry to keep you unhealthy and coming back for more. And in fact that's exactly what the ultraprocessed-food producers want.

Let's move on to another aspect of a typical day that exacerbates disconnection syndrome.

Breaking News Breaks the Brain

Some of us like to prepare for the day by informing ourselves of world events. Ninety-five percent of Americans say they follow the news, and 85 percent of us check the news at least once a day.[13] News is increasing stress and stimulating fight or flight — speaking directly to the amygdala and drawing attention away from the prefrontal cortex. Whether it's the unnerving breaking news headlines or the word *alert* constantly flashing on the bottom of the television screen, the nature of news delivery today breeds fear and anxiety and perpetuates a state of chronic stress. And it's not as though we're getting reliable information out of our news exposure, since only 22 percent of us trust our local news "a lot."[14] This number shrinks to 18 percent for national news organizations.[15] But among American adults relying on social media for news, only 4 percent trust the information they receive. In addition, we have little faith in a nonpartisan news system: 74 percent of us believe the news media is slanted toward one particular political party,[16] and 72 percent of us feel that the news "blows things out of proportion."[17] Given that we seem to view the news as one-sided and untrustworthy, maybe it's time to take the remote away from your stress-loving amygdala.

What happens when we start to view the world through the lens of chronic stress and fear and lose the rational, cool-headed prefrontal cortex? We see things in an unnecessarily negative way. Though we live in a time of relative peace and economic stability, with lower rates of extreme poverty and higher rates of democracy around the world than ever before, in 2017 more Americans than ever believed life was worse than it was fifty years earlier, during the heart of the Vietnam War.[18] Crime rates in the United States fell from the 1990s to the 2000s.[19] Despite this, many believed the opposite. Of those who felt crime was increasing, the top reasons cited for this belief were television and the newspapers.[20] One poll about the causes of American stressors showed that among those reporting "a great deal of stress," 40 percent cited news as a causative factor.[21] Only fifteen minutes of exposure to news was enough to increase symptoms of anxiety in college students.[22] And this relates directly to neuroplasticity: the more we dwell on negativity, the more our brains become primed for pessimism and, as such, the more we're inclined to view the world around us in a negative light. Through neuroplasticity, the more you experience negativity, the more negative you become.

Dr. Kalev Leetaru is a research scientist focusing on big-data analysis. He has been fondly called the "wizard of big data" by Georgetown University and is a senior fellow at the Center for Cyber and Homeland Security at Auburn University (formerly at George Washington University). He frequently writes about the ways we use data to understand the world. In 2011 he published a paper called "Culturomics 2.0," which reviewed the complete text of the *New York Times* between 1945 and 2005 (5.9 million articles) as well as English-language Web news from 2006 to 2011.[23] This fascinating review showed that the *New York Times,* according to Leetaru, "exhibits a strong decade-long trend towards negativity from the early 1960s to the early 1970s, before recovering towards slight negativity, and has trended slightly more negative in recent years up to the 11 September 2001 attacks, which caused news to become sharply more negative in the following four years."

Because there was concern that the *New York Times* may only be representative of trends in the United States, the study also reviewed data from a service called Summary of World Broadcasts and found "a steady, near linear, march towards negativity" from 1979 to 2010. Why does all this matter? Much of the negativity in modern news stems from political and ideological division. It comes from fear and anger, the emotions that promote amygdala activity. In this way, our exposure to negativity is perpetuating the bigger problem. In addition, while we can likely agree that living life in a constantly negative state is less than ideal, it's worth noting that negativity is associated with consistently worse health outcomes across a variety of conditions. Finally, more negativity may mean higher levels of the stress hormone cortisol. As you'll recall, stress turbocharges the amygdala.

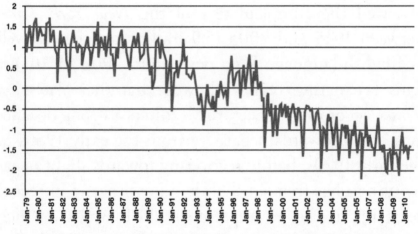

Average monthly tone of *Summary of World Broadcasts* news content, January 1979–July 2010.

Adapted from Dr. Kalev H. Leetaru's "Culturomics 2.0: Forecasting Large-scale Human Behavior Using Global News Media Tone in Time and Space," *First Monday* 16, no. 9 (2011). Reprinted with permission.

What's more, we now have to worry about false or purposely misleading news. A 2017 study conducted by MIT shows that false news "diffused significantly farther, faster, deeper, and more broadly than the truth in all categories."[24] False news was 70 percent more likely to be retweeted than true news. Interestingly, robotic spread of news was equivalent for both true and false news, implying that it's people—not bots—that are sharing the misinformation. And 86 percent of Americans reading articles on social media may skip fact-checking. More important, we're unable to distinguish real from false news. A recent study showed that despite 59 percent of young adults feeling "very confident" in their critical-thinking skills, the majority could not consistently tell the difference between fake news and real news.[25] That's not necessarily a criticism. These days, determining what is truly valid is a daunting task. And when we don't know what's true anymore, we fall victim to the sensationalizing and divisive stories that seem so common today. This activates fear and anger, again pushing us away from the ability to use our prefrontal cortices. Of course, with the rational prefrontal cortex offline, we're less likely to question the validity of the news, and our problem gets even worse.

Another concern is that news sites and other technologies hijack our reward circuit to steal our attention and time. Digital platforms (especially social media) use an algorithmic approach to determine what to show us. This results in filter bubbles—the outcome of computer programs that selectively choose what each of us sees when we go online. These algorithms are tasked with holding our attention, not improving our education or the quality of our lives. What we see on the computer screen is engineered to take something from us, extracting our data, attention, or money.

We're constantly exposed to salacious and hyperbolic Web links called clickbait. There's a reason clickbait is so pervasive and extreme: the goal is to keep us coming back for more. It's a dopamine button. And every time we click, we push the brain's buttons to feed amygdala-based responses that remove us further from the prefrontal cortex.

Workplace Woes

Once we make it to work, we're unhappy, distracted, and stressed. We find ourselves disconnected from our jobs. In fact, around half of Americans report dissatisfaction with their jobs.[26] Employees say they're bored with work for around ten hours a week,[27] and a Gallup survey found that 87 percent of employees worldwide are not engaged in their jobs.[28] It's no wonder, then, that 79 percent of American employees say they always, often, or sometimes are distracted or find it difficult to concentrate at work.[29] It's also no wonder that, disengaged and disconnected from work, we find it hard to bring the prefrontal cortex online to accomplish higher-level thinking. And, with distraction and stress levels so high, employees spend around five hours a week on their phones at work doing nonwork activities. They are seeking relief to no avail. And rather than doing something truly healthful—exercising, meditating, being out in nature—they are drawn to addictive behaviors, many of which are isolating and sedentary. As we'll later see, isolation and spending too much time sitting down or otherwise being inactive are dual villains in our lives.

The End of Days

After struggling through the day at work, our brains appear too fatigued to accomplish much. The average American spends nearly six hours a day watching media on TV, the computer, and mobile devices (of which four hours and forty-five minutes is TV time), meaning we tune in as soon as we get home.[30] We seek out a quick reward to relieve the stress of the day, and a high-carbohydrate, unhealthful meal does the trick. And, of course, we continue using our smartphones as we eat—scrolling, clicking, texting, constantly activating the reward circuit. This gives us the sense that we are somehow connected, when in reality we are deeply disconnected from what really matters most. We end our days hoping for a good night's sleep away from the day's obligations and stressors, but again, even that is an elusive goal.

As you can see, the typical day is filled with things that keep our amygdalas engaged and our prefrontal cortices inhibited. Moreover, modern life increasingly tempts us with the easy out when we're stressed out. We have constant access to short-term happiness and addictive rewards. Unfortunately, these make the problem worse. We have been brainwashed into believing that the way to lasting happiness is to double down on the very things that are making us miserable.

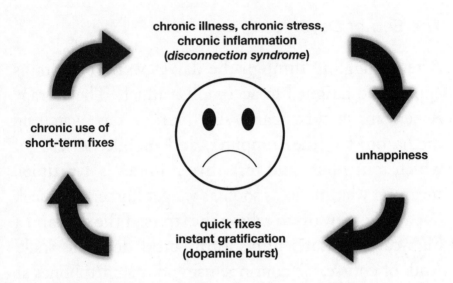

The good news is that your day is filled with opportunities to change for the better. To bring the brain's various functions into balance. To awaken that sedated prefrontal cortex and reconnect to it. Only then can we save ourselves and the planet.

CHAPTER 4

High-Tech Hijack

How Digital Life Disconnects

In a world where we are able to jump on an app to order dinner, get a ride from a stranger, or even pay our bills, there seems to be a decreasing need for human interactions. Technology is a tool that has allowed countless advances in medicine, psychology, industry, and more, but it's also allowing us to automate ourselves away from human connection and personal intimacy—creating more emotionally detached people than ever before in history.

—LISA STROHMAN, JD, PhD,
FOUNDER OF DIGITAL CITIZEN
ACADEMY

Technology is a useful servant but a dangerous master.

—CHRISTIAN LOUS LANGE, WINNER
OF THE NOBEL PEACE PRIZE

WHEN I (AUSTIN) WAS A child, I saw cell phones only in futuristic movies and TV shows. If I wanted to contact a friend, I used the family landline. The internet was a burgeoning world of information that we didn't really know what to do with. Encyclopedias and textbooks were still the go-to sources of information.

In the years to follow, personal technology would revolutionize communications. I went from AOL Instant Messenger and dial-up internet to Myspace and a flip phone. At the time, the benefits appeared substantial: if I was lost, I could call for help; if I was running late, I could text people and let them know. If I wanted to connect with distant friends, I could reach out.

When I started using social media, I saw so many possibilities. I could see what everyone in the world was doing without leaving the comfort of my couch. I could maintain friendships better. I could easily test an idea on a large scale and learn from an incredibly diverse group of humans across the world. But in practice, I would simply scroll mindlessly through photos and posts to kill time. I'd wade through ads, hateful comments, and semiformed thoughts. Social media became my biggest time sink and a powerful hindrance to productivity and personal growth. This isn't to say that social media can't have real benefits, but I was neglecting to ask the question: What is social media taking from me?

Phones, computers, and tablets have transitioned from objects that seemed explicitly designed to make life easier into attention-grabbing machines. I watched while my peers stopped using technology to improve their lives and started using it to *replace active living.* It's rare to go out to dinner or spend time with friends without having digital devices interfere with quality moments. I'm often part of a conversation that is fragmented by an incoming text or alert. Before I implemented the changes outlined in the Brain Wash program, my concentration was incessantly broken by an ongoing need to check my email, Facebook, or Instagram. This is not a healthy state of being.

DIGITAL DISTRACTION

There may be no aspect of the modern world that is more revolutionary or quickly evolving than technology. It is highly useful and facilitates a wide range of conveniences that make our lives better. Technological advances in every area—from medicine to manufacturing—have revolutionized society and allowed humans to thrive in ways that were previously unimaginable. Modern technology makes most areas of our lives easier, from shopping to work, travel, education, entertainment, banking, and communications. The spread of the internet and associated communication technologies has also helped democratize knowledge, providing free education to anyone with a computer, tablet, or smartphone in the form of podcasts, blogs, and YouTube videos. But we all know modern technology has its dark sides. There is no doubt that it distracts us. It activates our reward circuitry, luring us in with the addictive pull of instant gratification. Overreliance on new technologies also promotes mindless behavior. Too much aimless surfing and scrolling through online stores and social media leads us to wonder where our time and energy have gone. But remember, these websites want to set our minds adrift for hours on end.

Science is still figuring out how spending time on these mindless pursuits affects our mental health. But we do have some early answers, and we also know that as we increase the time spent on digital connection, we decrease the time spent on introspection and in-person interaction. The scale of this shift is massive and readily observable in any public setting. The focus of our waking hours is dramatically changed. This transition in our attention must be considered in the context of our overall goals. As we change our lives to foster long-term happiness and healthful decisions, our use of modern technology—and the way this changes our brains—must not be ignored.

Most of us are at the mercy of the internet and its temptations purely because we depend on it for work and many of the other daily activities of contemporary life. We are caught in limbo, trying to balance the positive and negative sides of technology in our lives. Technology has become essential in navigating the modern-day world, but it also exposes our minds to what are without a doubt the most advanced persuasive techniques ever developed. There's a good reason why it's so hard to put down our devices: they are designed to be addictive.

Tristan Harris is a former design ethicist at Google. He's also a veteran magician who likes to draw parallels between the ways in which magicians and product developers operate—i.e., by exploiting weaknesses in the human mind. He writes: "Magicians start by looking for blind spots, edges, vulnerabilities and limits of people's perception, so they can influence what people do without them even realizing it. Once you know how to push people's buttons, you can play them like a piano."[1]

What does it look like when modern technology uses this knowledge against us? We become captives of the dopamine that floods our brains every time we check a post for likes, repeatedly refresh our email in-boxes, or add an unnecessary purchase to our online shopping carts. This addictive power has been slow to make it into medical textbooks. Most of these technologies simply haven't been tested using valid scientific methods over the long term. They also haven't been around long enough for us to arrive at any certain conclusions. These are tricky areas to study. But despite these challenges, we're already beginning to document some striking medical issues. The best example to date may be internet addiction.

A NEW ADDICTION

Though internet addiction is not yet recognized as an official diagnosis by the standard psychiatric diagnostic manual (the *Diagnostic and Statistical Manual of Mental Disorders,* or DSM-5), it's nonetheless being increasingly treated as a real problem, and for good reason. An international meta-analysis found that rates of internet addiction—any online-related compulsive behavior that interferes with normal living and causes severe stress on family, friends, loved ones, and the ability to be productive at work—are around 6 percent.[2] This clearly qualifies as a disease state. With more than four billion internet users worldwide, that 6 percent translates to more than a quarter of a billion people whose level of internet usage and dependence qualify as an addiction.[3] That's close to five times the population of England. This number is likely to get a whole lot bigger, because some of the world's largest companies are trying to increase the addictive potential of our digital media.

It's important to point out that addiction per se is not the only concern here. We need to also focus on the problems that result from an addicted mind. The authors of the analysis we just mentioned found that internet addiction "is inversely associated with the quality of life, as reflected by both subjective (life satisfaction) and objective (quality of environmental conditions) indicators." Simply put, internet addiction is linked to low life satisfaction. This means there's more at play than the addiction. We can't just assume that the addiction caused the low life satisfaction. It could be that people who don't enjoy life are more likely to become internet addicts. Either way, this is a problem. Internet addiction rates may also be highest in young generations: results from a recent study in China show that rates of internet addiction among adolescents are much higher than the global average, at around 16 percent.[4] This is consistent with other studies, including those conducted in the United States, that reveal a culture of internet addiction among young folks who grew up with the internet.[5]

With these types of numbers, we have to ask: What is happening in the brain? In the last few years, researchers have helped answer this question. Multiple high-quality studies have demonstrated actual structural changes in the brains of internet-addicted individuals compared to healthy controls.[6] One area in particular is called the anterior cingulate, a region of the brain that has a unique connection to both the limbic brain and the prefrontal cortex. Alongside the prefrontal cortex, it helps moderate impulse control. It's concerning, then, that research has clearly revealed that the anterior cingulate is smaller in size among internet addicts than it is in other people. One recent study showed that internet addicts may also have weaker connections between their prefrontal cortices and their anterior cingulates.[7]

We aren't yet sure if people with these brain characteristics are more likely to become internet addicts or if internet addiction causes these characteristics, but we do know that our choices and actions change our brains. If there is even a small chance that overuse of addictive technology triggers these structural differences, we need to take these results seriously. Anyone who uses the internet is vulnerable to some degree to its effects on the brain. In other words, *you don't have to qualify as an internet addict to suffer the consequences.*

Mind Less

Beyond the effects on our addiction circuitry, technology can disconnect us from our high-level brains by promoting mindless activity. Our ability to be thoughtful, focused, and present gets squandered when we turn our attention to clickbait, an endless scroll through newsfeeds, or an unbroken video queue. When we finally snap out of the nearly unconscious state in which we pursue these activities, we realize how much time has vanished and how little we have to show for it—certainly nothing productive. Our brains might as well have been hibernating. And once we realize how much time we've lost, we can start to feel annoyed and down on ourselves, driving our brains to seek a quick fix and perpetuating that vicious cycle. It's easy to see how we then find ourselves starting another episode or heading to the kitchen for some junk food.

It's crucial to understand that your mindless state benefits corporations, since it keeps you from questioning the use of your time. The longer you spend on a website, app, or other digital platform, the better for its owners' revenue. This is why YouTube has autoplay, a built-in feature that automatically plays a related video based on your viewing history, and why websites are willing to post egregiously hyperbolic clickbait. We'll show you an easy and practical way to combat this mindless behavior at the end of the chapter.

Friend Less

Though there are definite benefits to be gained from digital communication, we know that it's not the same as in-person interaction. And increasingly, we see that our digital devices are getting in the way of quality time spent together in the nondigital world. They distract us and damage our relationships.

In one 2018 study, several hundred people were recruited to share a meal at a restaurant with friends or family members.[8] Some participants left their phones on the table while others stored them away. Unsurprisingly, those who left their phones out reported more distraction and lower enjoyment of the meal. Having a phone present during a conversation between two strangers (even when it didn't belong to either of them) was linked in another study to lower levels of perceived empathic concern.[9] When the phone was taken away, the strangers reported "significantly superior" interactions. These studies are a pointed reminder to put away your phone during your next meal or conversation.

A study conducted by researchers at the University of Chicago and Harvard showed that shaking hands with another person increases cooperative behavior and improves outcomes in negotiations.[10] This is just one way we benefit from the wealth of information and nuance that come from in-person engagement. Body language, facial expressions, and even the smell of another person all contribute to the complex interplay in face-to-face communication. Much of this is lost when we go digital.

The shared space of digital life is "disembodied space," as Stephen Asma aptly describes it. A philosopher and coauthor of *The Emotional Mind,* Asma points out the chief shortfalls of the digital world: "We cannot really touch one another, smell one another, detect facial expressions or moods, and so on. Real bonding is more biological than psychological and requires physical contact. The emotional entanglement of real friendship produces oxytocin and endorphins in the brains and bodies of friends—cementing them together in ways that are more profound than other relationships."[11]

Dr. Lisa Strohman, a psychologist and expert in technology wellness, echoed this sentiment when we spoke with her: "The simple art of behavioral cues that we pick up in person when someone is leaning into our conversation, blushing at a comment, or even shifting in her seat is all lost when we rely solely on technological exchanges. We encode our memories through our senses: the smell of the grass when we had our first kiss, the comfort from a warm cup of hot chocolate, or even the familiar sounds of the birds from your childhood home are all sensory inputs that bring us front and center to an emotional space we encode into a permanent memory. As we fall into this digital world and learn to live without these emotional connections, we lose part of what makes us social beings interconnected through humanity, grace, and love."[12]

Mental Well Less

The overuse of modern technology also correlates with the presence of mental health issues. In a 2017 paper that reviewed trials relating to smartphone usage and mental health among adults, one pattern was documented repeatedly: depression, anxiety, and stress were all tied to problematic smartphone use.[13] "Problematic" in this context means excessive—using a smartphone so much that it interferes with life. College students who use the internet very frequently also have repeatedly been found to experience depressive symptoms. More disturbing, a review of available studies has shown that internet addiction in adults is associated with almost double the risk of suicide and nearly *quadruple* the risk in those under the age of eighteen.[14] Again, this is only association. We don't know whether people with depression are more likely to overuse modern technology or if it's the other way around. The results are nonetheless striking.

There are many reasons why young people may be particularly vulnerable to these effects. First, they're the top users of these new technologies. Second, their minds are still developing and are therefore more malleable. With these concerns in mind, pediatricians have finally chimed in on the growing digital problem. In 2018 their flagship journal, *Pediatrics,* published a paper in which the authors describe a "normalized addiction" to social media use in particular, explaining that "usage patterns among adolescents resemble the progressive, withdrawal-producing and dose-dependent symptoms of substance addiction."[15]

Because of this potent addictive tendency, they recommend that health-care providers ask a set of questions to all adolescents over the age of eleven to determine whether social media use is a significant problem in their lives. Sample questions include "Do you think you use social media too much?" and "Does viewing social media increase or decrease your self-confidence?"

If you think this is extreme, consider that across Asia, far more aggressive interventions have been put in place. In China, boot camps have been established for social-media-addicted teenagers, and South Korean children are similarly finding themselves at digital detox facilities that emphasize human interaction in hopes of "rebuilding connections back to the real world," since many of them "only have online friends."[16] Even if these examples don't particularly apply to you or your loved ones, all of us need to take heed. When it comes to digital exposure, children may be the canaries in the coal mine. And there may be no aspect of our modern technology as popular or as problematic as social media—for both kids and adults.

> "When you've got five minutes to fill, Twitter is a great way to fill thirty-five minutes."
> —Matt Cutts, software engineer and former head of Google's Web spam team[17]

Social Disconnection

We are social creatures. We need one another to survive. That's partly why we so strongly gravitate to social technologies like Facebook and Instagram: social media allows us to come together to share ideas and love, regardless of location. But this comes at a cost. And when we consider the scope of social media engagement, any negative impact is of global concern.

On average, people around the world who use the internet have 8.5 social media accounts.[18] Predictably, people between the ages of sixteen and twenty-four are are devoting the most time per day to social media— three hours and one minute, on average. By contrast, people between the ages of fifty-five and sixty-four are maintaining 2.85 accounts. Let's put the numbers into context by first considering the total worldwide population: 7.7 billion people. By the time you read this it could be close to eight billion. As previously noted, the internet has more than four billion users, and there are 3.5 billion active social media users. The average time spent on social media is two hours and twenty-two minutes.[19]

SOCIAL MEDIA MADNESS IN THE UNITED STATES IN 2018[20]

- 88% of 18- to 29-year-olds use some form of social media

- 78% of 30- to 49-year-olds use some form of social media

- 68% of adults use Facebook

- 74% of Facebook users visit the site daily

- 35% of adults use Instagram, a 7% increase from 2017

- 78% of 18- to 24-year-olds use Snapchat, and 71% of them use the app several times a day

- 41% of women use Pinterest

Do you feel like you use social media in a way that adds meaning and value to your life? Or does it impede your ability to live life to the fullest? Some of the people closest to the development of social media have started to ask this question. Their perspectives are quite eye-opening.

Chamath Palihapitiya is a venture capitalist who was involved with the creation of Facebook, a company he left in 2011. In an interview at the Stanford Graduate School of Business, he was asked about his role in helping create the social media enterprise, and he responded honestly: "I feel tremendous guilt. I think we knew something bad could happen." He went on to say that "we have created tools that are ripping apart the social fabric of how society works" and that "people need to hard break from some of these tools."[21]

Sadly, there's not much evidence that we're taking his message to heart. Social media use is on the rise—so much so that a team of researchers calculated how much someone would have to be paid to walk away from Facebook for a year. Dr. Jay Corrigan, a professor of economics at Kenyon College, led the study using a series of auctions in which people were paid to close their accounts for as little as one day or as long as one year. Dr. Corrigan's team, in collaboration with researchers at Tufts University and Michigan State University, found that Facebook users would require an average of more than $1,000 to deactivate their accounts for one year.[22] Apparently, we love our social media so much that we have to be paid to sign off!

Another study encompassed more than a thousand people who were using Facebook with regularity (94 percent of the participants reported using Facebook as part of a daily routine, and most of those used it for thirty minutes or more a day).[23] The researchers chose certain individuals at random who would continue using Facebook as usual, then asked the others to stop using the site for one week. Participants were asked questions about their quality of life both before and after the study. Those who abstained for the week reported a significantly higher level of life satisfaction than those using it as usual. Perhaps unsurprisingly, those who stayed off the site also reported an increase in satisfaction with their social lives in the real world compared to those still using Facebook.

A similar experiment was conducted by researchers at the University of Pennsylvania, where 143 undergraduates were assigned to either limit their use of Facebook, Instagram, and Snapchat to ten minutes per platform per day or use the apps as usual for three weeks.[24] The researchers monitored screenshots showing how many minutes a day were spent on the various applications. After the intervention, people with limited social media use scored significantly lower on a scale of loneliness. Those in the limited-social-media group who had high depression scores at the start of the experiment had lower depression scores at the end.

In another study, researchers conducted a survey of almost 1,800 Americans between the ages of nineteen and thirty-two.[25] They examined their social media use in relation to the degree of social isolation they felt. Results showed that those who used social media the most had more than three times the rate of social isolation than those who used it least had. The study concluded by saying, "Contrary to our hypothesis, young adults with high social media use seem to be more, and not less, socially isolated."

We are not trying to say that social media doesn't have its benefits. It is a powerful tool for business, global engagement, and interpersonal support. But we need to understand that the impact of passive, mindless use of social media may be completely different from that of active, engaged use. Social media serves us far better when we use it *with purpose*. There's data to prove this point.[26] When we actively engage in social media — posting and commenting in positive communication with others rather than passively scrolling and just looking at posts — we may benefit and avoid the pitfalls that we've been describing. But therein lies the challenge: how to strike the balance between healthful use and unhealthful use. We'll outline steps to help you with this shortly, but for now, start to think about how and why you're using social media, then ask yourself whether what you're doing is helping you or simply filling a void. Consider setting a timer for five minutes next time you go on a social media platform, and when the clock runs out, ask yourself what you're hoping to gain from further use. Is this the best use of your time? If not, sign off. This is a simple exercise, but it may be revealing.

Earlier we explained that internet addiction is linked

to structural changes in the brain. Given that unhealthful social media engagement could be seen as a form of internet addiction, it should come as no surprise that scientists have documented such changes specifically as a result of social media usage. Neuroimaging studies show that people who use social media excessively (to the point of developing addictive tendencies) have less white matter in the corpus callosum—the part of the brain connecting the left and right hemispheres.[27] This means these twin halves may be less efficiently connected. People who have a genetic malformation of this important connection often have difficulties with social interaction and learning. Indeed, it's paradoxical that by engaging in excessive social media use we may well be simultaneously damaging our ability to authentically interact with others.

This directly ties in to our sense of self-worth. We're all vulnerable to social approval—the need to belong, to be accepted and appreciated by our peers, is among the highest human motivators. Again, this goes back to our primal need to connect with and be accepted in a tribe just to survive. But now our social approval is in the hands of tech companies. In 2016, Dr. Lauren Sherman and her colleagues at the University of California at Los Angeles used functional MRI to study the ways in which the brain is affected by social media.[28] She and her team exposed adolescents to images that were reported to be from Instagram, then changed the number of "likes" seen on the individual photos. The study found that, not unexpectedly, photos with the most likes appeared to increase activation in the parts of the brain involved in reward pathways. A later study showed that liking photos also lit up these brain areas. Is it any wonder we're so hooked?[29]

And here is the real issue: you think you're playing the game the right way—the way everyone else does—by buying into the social platform. Humans feel safest doing what others do, so we think our engagement with these platforms is harmless. Meanwhile, your reward circuit is being manipulated every time someone interacts with your posts. Your reward system is being hacked right in front of you. You are the one being played.

Technology has always been essential to our survival and success as a species. The creation of fire required new technology. The spoon was at one point a novel technological invention. Many aspects of our modern tech are also incredibly helpful. We have to appreciate, however, that we've reached a new point in our evolution, one where technology is able to use and manipulate us. We also cannot ignore the fact that we've become inextricably tethered to our devices to the exclusion of meaningful, in-person interactions. Moreover, technology tends to expose us to artificial light—notably, blue light—which will hinder other aspects of a healthy life, such as getting sound sleep (see chapter 8). And, most important, we have to address the fact that our digital interactions may be adversely changing our brains.

Our mission in this book is to give you back the

power to think clearly and the ability to make the choices that benefit you best in the long run. Addictive, mindless, distracting tech — some of which will just bring you down emotionally — keeps you from reaching that goal. But whether your problem is social media, video bingeing, email fatigue, or just unhealthful internet use in general, we have a tool for you.

DOES IT PASS THE TEST OF T.I.M.E.?

Apps have started to emerge to help people track their screen time and avoid smartphone addiction. But you don't need an app for this exercise. You can go low-tech here and use our T.I.M.E. tool. When approaching your use of technology, especially when it comes to digital media and communication, you need to make sure your activities are making good use of T.I.M.E. This means they need to be...

Time restricted. Create and abide by a minimum window of time for accomplishing your goals. If you want to watch YouTube videos or scroll through a social media platform — but you often spend more time than you'd like doing so — set a timer to go off after twenty minutes. If, after checking in with friends or buying essentials online, you find yourself aimlessly scrolling through online shopping sites, set a five- or ten-minute timer for these activities. Continue tweaking your timer until you've found the right spot, and respect the clock!

Intentional. As we've described in detail, so much of our interaction with technology is designed to benefit others. Becoming more intentional about our use of digital products helps put the power back in your hands. Before engaging with email, social media, videos, TV, or any other personally problematic technology, ask yourself what you're hoping to get out of it and whether it is truly something that benefits you. If you find that you can't come up with acceptable answers to these questions, rethink your plan. Be intentional with every digital action.

Mindful. A mindful approach to digital media consumption means bringing awareness to the way you're using these technologies while you're using them as well as awareness of the way they are affecting you. This type of conscious digital use counters the trap created by mindless activity. What does this look like in practice? Try incorporating pauses into your digital consumption during which you question the way you're using the technology and the way it's making you feel. Is a website making you angry? Does scrolling through a photo feed make you feel self-conscious, envious, inadequate, or inferior? Mindfulness grants you a window into your brain and gives you the opportunity to pull back if you don't like what you see.

* * *

Enriching. The digital sphere is filled with clickbait and other content designed to capture your attention. Much of this is a waste of your time. But digital media also gives us access to an incredible wealth of knowledge, helping us better understand ourselves and our world. The way to separate these two disparate experiences is to ask yourself whether what you're taking in is enriching. Does it add to your knowledge? Better you as a person? Make you feel more content and optimistic? Or is it just a distraction?

Give everything you do the test of T.I.M.E.!

CHAPTER 5

The Gift of Empathy

Freedom from Disconnection Syndrome

Yet, taught by time, my heart has learned to glow
For others' good, and melt at others' woe.

—Homer

No man is an island, entire of itself; every man is a piece of
the continent.

—John Donne

MANY YEARS AGO, WHILE I (David) was making hospital rounds, seeing patients, I went into the room of a gentleman who was recovering from a stroke. Frank was improving nicely, but then he began to experience some setbacks that prolonged his hospital stay. While we were chatting, I noticed that his mood had shifted dramatically since my previous visit. Perhaps it was because he began to realize that his life was forever changed by the event in his brain, or maybe he had just been in the hospital too long. Nonetheless, he was down.

As we were talking, I mentioned his mood change. As I recall, he looked at the floor and shook his head, telling me, "I'm not happy anymore." I asked what I could do to help and suggested that we arrange to get him outside for a bit. I will never forget his response: "All I want is an onion sandwich."

I paused. First, I was puzzled that something like an onion sandwich could play such a pivotal role in this man's mood, and second, I didn't even know what an onion sandwich was! I asked, "What's an onion sandwich?" And he explained that it was simply a thick slice of onion on white bread with mayonnaise.

Okay, that was easy. I asked him why this would make him happy. He explained that when he was a child, whenever he was upset, his mother would make him an onion sandwich. Obviously, this was a deep-seated memory, and it offered up a terrific opportunity for me to help my patient.

After we visited for a few more minutes, I went out to the nurses' station and asked if we could put an onion sandwich on Frank's menu for lunch. They checked with the hospital kitchen staff, who reported back that this wasn't something on the "normal menu," so I was refused.

Knowing how important this was for Frank, I was not about to be deterred. I took up his chart and opened it to the section where doctors order tests, medications, and other items. I specifically wrote an order for an onion sandwich, spelling out in detail exactly how it should be made.

I then saw the rest of my patients and returned to my office.

The next morning was busy, because I had several new patients to admit to the hospital. After I was finished, I made my rounds, and by the time I came to Frank's room, I wasn't thinking about my visit with him the day before. When I walked into his room, he had a big smile on his face. I can't say for sure whether it was the onion sandwich, but Frank's condition had improved so rapidly that I was able to discharge him the next day.

A little compassion goes a long way. Trouble is, modern culture drives us toward self-serving behaviors. Would Frank get an onion sandwich today? As we've said, humans are an inherently social species, and many of our most brilliant successes — as a society and even as individuals — come from teamwork and collaboration. To navigate the world effectively, we must be able to understand and care about the actions and even thoughts and beliefs of others. We must support our empathic capabilities if we are to free ourselves from the grip of disconnection syndrome and find true happiness. It's time we realize that what's best for me is what's best for we.

> It is our interconnectedness, our interrelationships, not just among people but also among all living things, that sustains us and provides resilience against adversity. Unfortunately, our brains are progressively reinforced to believe that we are the center of the universe and that getting ahead requires others to falter and fail.

EMPATHY EXPLAINED

Most parents have had the experience of tending to a child in distress without a second thought. You're sitting in a chair reading an engrossing book when your toddler suddenly falls down while playing nearby, scrapes her knee, and starts to cry. Your attention is immediately diverted from the story you've been reading, and you quickly attend to your daughter, whose distress you perceive almost unconsciously. You understand what she feels and actively want to comfort her.

According to Jean Decety and Philip L. Jackson, in their beautiful paper entitled "The Functional Architecture of Human Empathy," this natural, virtually magical ability "to understand the emotions and feeling of others, whether one actually witnessed his or her situation, perceived it from a photograph, read about it in [a] fiction book, or merely imagined it, refers to the phenomeno-logical experience of empathy."[1] Professor William Ickes of the University of Texas at Arlington, a longtime researcher on empathy, calls it "everyday mind-reading."[2] And for good reason: *empathic inference*—asking questions in your head such as "What does she want?" "How does he feel about that?" "What are they trying to accomplish?"—is a part of the brain's hardware that usually comes preinstalled, although, as we will soon see, it is also something that can be cultivated. The basic building blocks are there at birth and develop through our inter-actions with others.

Empathic inference has its roots in our evolutionary past. As our brains developed and grew more sophisti-cated, we shaped and honed neural networks to help us rapidly evaluate the motivations of others, work together to gather and hunt for food, detect the pres-ence of predators, and ensure successful reproduction through courtship and social intelligence. While vari-ous kinds of empathy may be seen in other animals, only in humans is empathy a complex form of psycho-logical inference that involves multiple mental pro-cesses: feeling what another person is feeling, knowing what another person is feeling, and wanting to respond compassionately to another person's distress.

In this book we will focus on two major types of empathy. The first type, called *affective empathy,* gives us the ability to experience the emotions of others. This is why we wince when we watch someone stub her toe.

It's why we leap toward hurt children. We "feel their pain." Many cognitive neuroscientists and neuropsychologists believe that so-called mirror neurons, which are neurons that fire both when you act and when you watch someone else perform that same act, help us learn new skills by imitation, though this theory has fallen out of favor in recent years. We do know that our brains are set up to allow us to share in the experiences of others. We just aren't sure exactly how it happens yet.

The second type of empathy is called *cognitive empathy,* also known as "theory of mind" or "perspective-taking." This is the ability to see things from the perspective of another—to understand the motives of others and to be consciously aware of their thoughts, intentions, and desires. It is the ability to put yourself in someone else's shoes or, more precisely, in someone else's thinking brain. It's wonderful but potentially challenging to appreciate alternative viewpoints. Unfortunately, in our polarized, feverishly partisan world, examples of cognitive empathy are increasingly hard to find. But this type of empathy can absolutely be cultivated and enhanced.

With this understanding of empathy, the concept of narcissism becomes easy to define. Narcissism is a deficit of empathy—a lack of focus on or caring about others. It involves a sense of entitlement and a hyperfocus on oneself. It's important to understand that the fundamental characteristics of narcissism are low empathy, high selfishness, disregard for others, and self-centeredness. Two types of narcissism are often described. One type may prove advantageous because it encompasses a set of personality traits involving high self-esteem, which can translate to a high likelihood of career success. But because this trait also involves low empathy, interpersonal relationships can suffer. The second is the "clinical" type, involving a fixed and inflexible pattern of delusions of self-importance and uniqueness, a pervasive pattern of grandiosity, an excessive need for admiration, and a total lack of empathy. This is known as narcissistic personality disorder. Other personality disorders can also include narcissistic behaviors. Right now, we bet you can think of at least one person in your life—whom you know personally, professionally, or through media—that you could label as mildly or severely narcissistic.

University of Michigan researcher Dr. Sara Konrath has shown that students who went to college after the year 2000 have much lower empathy levels than those who came before them. Dr. Konrath writes, "College kids today are about 40 percent lower in empathy than their counterparts of 20 or 30 years ago, as measured by standard tests of this personality trait."[3]

Why should we be more empathic and less narcissistic? How does empathy benefit us? The straight answer, supported by science, is that high levels of empathy are associated with life satisfaction, rich social networks, healthy relationships, heightened workplace performance, and greater overall well-being.[4] We're less adversely aggressive and more prosocial (friendly) and generous. Empathy paves the way for greater respect for the common good—respect for one's neighbors, community, country, society, and planet. When we can care for others to the extent that we can appreciate or even adopt their points of view, we stand to gain so much.

THE POSITIVE EFFECTS OF EMPATHY

Empathy may benefit us in a multitude of ways:

- Heightened feelings of trust, creativity, and compassion.

- Lower levels of stress (and, in turn, inflammation).

- Improved perception of others and an ability to relate, connect, and bond.

- Improved regulation of emotions and the capacity to combat struggles and frustrations.

- Heightened appreciation for the world around us, nature included.

Think of empathy as an important muscle in the body. When used regularly, it keeps your entire body strong, ready to perform, and running smoothly. And, like any muscle, it can be developed through specific exercises.

On the flip side, science shows that narcissism is related to domestic violence, sexual coercion, aggression, and offensive behavior directed toward others.[5] Research also finds that there's a strong correlation between levels of narcissism and the acceptance of violence by both men and women.[6] Which invites an important question: are violent and disrespectful acts toward certain groups of people in our society attributable in some part to blatant narcissism?

Narcissistic tendencies are hardly new. As Dr. W. Keith Campbell, a nationally recognized expert on narcissism, explains in a review of the literature, this trait is associated with "being liked in initial interactions…perceived as exciting…socially confident…entertaining…and able to obtain sexual partners."[7] Dr. Campbell, head of the department of psychology at the University of Georgia, studies the ways in which our culture is changing and what role narcissism and individualism play. He has a lot to say about social media. According to him, social media seems like it was perfectly designed to foster narcissism, because "narcissists function well in the context of shallow (as opposed to emotionally deep and committed) relationships." And Sacred Heart University's Dr. David G. Taylor, in a 2016 paper, found that "social media have provided an ideal platform for expressing one's sense of being special or exceptional."[8] So we have to ask ourselves: What does the following chart tell us?

Smartphone Apps Used Most Frequently

Apps	Number of Participants Using App (%)
Social networking sites	87%
Instant messaging	52%
News	51%
Gaming	25%
Shopping	21%
Music	19%
Photo/video apps	12%
TV catch-up	3%
Dating	2%
Fitness/diet	0.7%
Other	8%

Adapted from C. Pearson et al., *International Journal of Cyber Behavior, Psychology and Learning*. January–March 2015.

The vast majority of people using apps are doing so for social media purposes. Granted, social media—when it's a place for real connection and active interaction—can foster empathy. For example, if you're spending your time engaging honestly with those who are facing challenges in life, you're not going to get the result you would if you were actively seeking confirmation of your own greatness or comparing yourself to others. But can social media breed narcissism? Recent studies show this may well be the case. A 2018 paper was one of the first to suggest that excessive use of social media can increase narcissistic tendencies.[9] The researchers identified young people who were basically digitally dependent. The scientists' work indicated that when these individuals used Facebook and Instagram, there was a significant increase in their narcissistic traits after just a few months. They also noted that narcissism was significantly enhanced in individuals with low self-esteem. As we mentioned in the previous chapter, chronically comparing ourselves to others is a setup for low self-image, which in turn fuels narcissism. It's a vicious cycle.

Posting may be at its most narcissistic when involving the selfie. In 2019, Instagram reported that more than 400 million photos had the hashtag #selfie.[10] One survey calculated that the average millennial may take as many as 25,700 selfies during his or her lifetime and spend more than one hour each week taking selfies.[11]

It may not just be social media that we need to worry about. Another study looked at 565 college students and compared time they spent watching television to their scores on the Narcissistic Personality Inventory (a standardized test for determining levels of narcissism). Daily television watching, especially watching reality TV and political talk shows, was associated with narcissism.[12] The authors suggest that "television is one aspect of culture that may be responsible for cultivating greater narcissism in college students."

To be sure, these studies are correlative, not causative. Watching TV and engaging in social media will not necessarily cause you to become narcissistic. But these are important correlations we cannot ignore.

Millennials dedicate one hour per week to taking selfies, and it is estimated that they will take more than twenty-five thousand selfies in their lifetimes.

YOUR BRAIN ON EMPATHY

Empathy and narcissism are complex qualities and have been linked to multiple areas of the brain, including the prefrontal cortex, the amygdala, and others. In a 2018 study at the University of Nebraska, people with known damage to their prefrontal cortices were placed in conditions that tested their empathy.[13] The study found that they were less likely than those without such damage to give money to those who are suffering. There's also evidence that a weakened prefrontal cortex is linked to narcissism. A 2016 Chinese study looked at 176 college students and found that narcissism was related to decreased cortical thickness and decreased volume in the prefrontal cortex.[14] This confirms what science was beginning to understand in the mid-nineteenth century, when Phineas Gage's industrial accident severed connections within his prefrontal cortex.

Narcissism is a symptom of disconnection syndrome. In chapter 3, we discussed the role of chronic stress and cortisol in separating the prefrontal cortex from the amygdala and the fact that this may make us more impulsive and emotionally reactive. It also turns out that the stress-response systems of narcissists may be exceptionally sensitive to negative emotions. One study found that people high on the narcissism scale had significantly higher levels of cortisol in response to negative emotions than those with low levels of narcissism.[15] In another study, men with narcissistic tendencies were found to have significantly higher levels of baseline cortisol than those without narcissistic tendencies.[16] If our goal is to activate the prefrontal cortex so that we can make healthful decisions and live a life full of purpose, we need to think about this data closely and prioritize stress management.

While we're still learning much about the specific brain pathways involved in empathy and narcissism, there is another important finding to note. If, as researchers suggest, narcissists are constantly trying to "protect the grandiose self" from outside threats, then narcissists' fear mechanism may be overactive. This led researchers to an almost predictable conclusion: "In the context of narcissism, the amygdala may also play a vital role."[17]

We've learned much from brain-imaging studies about empathy and narcissism. For example, brain activation patterns change depending on the beneficiaries of our actions. In 2016, researchers at the University of Oxford, led by Dr. Patricia Lockwood, published a study in the journal *Proceedings of the National Academy of Sciences*.[18] In their clever experiment, the researchers scanned participants using an MRI machine while the participants carried out tasks. The specific tasks were based on scientifically validated models that test the ways in which people learn to reward themselves. Participants had to work out which symbols they needed to press to bring the biggest reward. In a twist, the participants also had to learn which symbols were more likely to give someone *else* a reward.

The results showed that people learned to reward themselves faster than they learned to help others. The team pinpointed the region of the brain that was activated when participants carried out actions that helped other people: the anterior cingulate, which, as we know, is associated with the prefrontal cortex, the amygdala, and the reward system. When the participants were learning how to help others, a specific part of the anterior cingulate was activated. This implies that the anterior cingulate is involved in controlling and regulating generosity.

Interestingly, the team also found that the anterior cingulate was not equally active in each of the scanned brains. Those who self-reported high levels of empathy had high activation levels, whereas individuals who rated themselves as less empathic had lower activation levels. Although previous studies have highlighted certain overlapping areas of the brain involved in empathy and prosocial behavior, this study adds a new level of specificity. In the words of Dr. Lockwood, "This is the first time anyone has shown a particular brain process for learning prosocial behaviors—and a possible link from empathy to learning to help others. By understanding what the brain does when we do things for other people, and interpersonal differences in this ability, we are better placed to understand what is going wrong in those whose psychological conditions are characterized by antisocial disregard for others."

Additional studies have confirmed similar findings, though we should reiterate that other areas of the brain also influence our empathic behaviors.[19] And as you might expect, there are genetic factors at play in this intricate system. A 2017 study showed that performing kind acts for others changes gene expression in a brain region involved in immune cell expression.[20] In other words, generosity may boost the immune system. And it may do so with the help of those reward pathways. (This is important: you can choose to activate your reward pathways for good!) In late 2018, similar research funded by the National Institutes of Health, which studied MRIs of people who gave to charities, revealed that generosity stimulates the reward center in the brain.[21] Such stimulation releases a flood of feel-good chemicals that strengthen the immune system. How so? Some of those feel-good chemicals, notably endorphins, seek out sick-looking cells and exert a healing effect on them.

This discovery is aligned with work conducted by Dr. Robert Waldinger, a psychiatrist and Harvard Medical School professor as well as the director of the world's longest-running study on happiness—the Harvard Study of Adult Development.[22] In his studies on happiness as people age, one of his most salient findings is that nurturing relationships strongly support our overall health and longevity. According to him, "Our relationships and how happy we are in our relationships has a powerful influence on our health." His studies have revealed that close relationships—more than money or fame—are what keep people happy throughout their lives. And those bonds are better predictors of a long and happy life than social class, IQ, and even inherited genetic influences. They protect us from life's discontents and help stave off mental and physical decline. We'll delve further into the power of relationships at the end of the book, but we bring it up here because there's no such thing as authentic bonding without empathy. We need to leverage the power of empathy to guard ourselves against disconnection syndrome.

In addition to brain wiring and its effect on empathic versus narcissistic tendencies, we need to mention the role of inflammation. One Japanese study tested the blood of its participants for a marker of low-grade inflammation called IL-6 (interleukin 6).[23] The researchers then asked participants questions to test their levels of comfort with economic inequality. Those with high levels of this inflammatory marker were more comfortable tolerating this inequality than those with low levels of this marker. That is to say, high levels of inflammation correlated with being less concerned about the problems of other people.

The strategies we offer in this book, and especially in the ten-day plan, will work to calm inflammation and reinforce the connections in the brain that let empathy rule. These strategies include everything from ramping up your empathic actions to improving your diet, increasing time spent in nature, engaging in mindfulness and meditation, and even practicing gratitude and volunteering (yes, the simple act of volunteering is associated with increased brain activity in the prefrontal cortex and anterior cingulate and, as a result, has been shown to correlate with improved executive function). On the other hand, you'll dial back things that diminish your empathic capabilities, such as the amount of time you spend comparing yourself to others and seeking validation on social media and online in general. You'll also reduce your consumption of foods that induce inflammation.

There's one more way that increased empathy can make a big impact in your life. Consider, for a moment, the short-term decisions you make that tend to harm you in the future. Poor food choices, binge-watching TV at the expense of adequate sleep, and repeatedly skipping exercise do little to help your future self. Thinking about that future version of you as another person—someone you need to look out for—puts empathy into play for your long-term benefit. We all need to start treating our future selves more kindly, looking out for their best interests through the choices we make today. Though it may sound somewhat silly at first, try putting yourself in the shoes of your future self, then tailoring your decisions to improve that person's quality of life. You won't regret it.

A TEACHABLE MOMENT

We seem to want to instill the values of empathy in our children. We teach them to share and to think about other people's feelings, asking them questions such as "How would you like it if that happened to you?" When children get into fights, we tell them to consider their impact on others and to choose their words carefully. Why do we forget to apply these concepts to our adult selves? Is empathy teachable and relearnable?

There may be no group of people for whom this question is more important than medical professionals. As doctors, we train in an environment of chronic and at times intense stress within a system that rewards us for doing better than our colleagues. It's no wonder that empathy dramatically declines during medical training. But we doctors have even more reason, beyond the general benefits of empathy already discussed, to care about this attribute. Empathic physicians get better patient compliance and better health outcomes. This makes good intuitive sense — patients want their doctors to care about them as people and not just as cases. When you feel a real connection with your physician, you're more likely to listen to his or her recommendations and follow his or her advice.

Researchers have taken an interest in trying to see whether medical professionals could be taught empathy. Thankfully, the answer appears to be yes. For example, a 2002 study hospitalized healthy second-year medical students for more than a day so they could experience health care from a patient's perspective.[24] They came away with what seemed to be a much better understanding of what things look like from the other side. Exposing health-care providers to a mindfulness technique called mindfulness-based stress reduction may also help increase empathy. More typical interventions, such as communications workshops, also appear to be effective in increasing empathy. In fact, a review of seventeen studies on teaching empathy to medical students concluded that "educational interventions can be effective in maintaining and enhancing empathy in undergraduate medical students."[25]

So interventions meant to enhance empathy are feasible and successful. However, we don't need research to tell us that. Just listening to the opinions of people with open minds, for example, will grant you insight into their views of the world. You'll then be better able to understand where they are coming from.

Empathy holds us together as families, communities, and societies. It can be cultivated—we outline ways to do so in the chapters ahead.

PART II

BREAKING THE SPELL

CHAPTER 6

It's Not Man Versus Nature

Getting Back to Our Roots

The best remedy for those who are afraid, lonely, or unhappy is to go outside, somewhere where they can be quite alone with the heavens, nature, and God.

—ANNE FRANK

In every walk with nature one receives far more than he seeks.

—JOHN MUIR

IN 1909, ENGLISH WRITER E. M. Forster wrote a disturbing short story entitled "The Machine Stops."[1] It painted a dark picture of the future, describing a world in which people spend their lives in isolated underground chambers, communicating with one another through digital devices that bear an uncanny resemblance to modern-day smartphones and tablets. In this dystopian future, humans worship the Machine, which controls all aspects of society, providing everything necessary for survival but stymieing in-person communication and exposure to nature. Indeed, the citizens of this fictional world are so removed from nature that they fear even the touch of sunlight upon their skin. As you might expect, this leads to catastrophe, and as the Machine collapses, the story's characters realize the grievous error they made in disconnecting from nature.

We aren't quite as lost as the characters in E. M. Forster's tale, but the parallels are obvious. More recently, the late Oliver Sacks reminded us of the Machine in an essay for *The New Yorker* that caught our attention.[2] We're increasingly separating ourselves from the natural world, spending a diminishing amount of time benefiting from its gifts. But our connection to nature is critical and plays a huge role in combating disconnection syndrome. Nature influences our ability to experience balance, thoughtfulness, and compassion while providing a panoply of health benefits, including reduced levels of inflammation and stress hormones. At a time when disconnection syndrome is becoming the status quo, we need to reconnect with the natural world around us— it's the original source of wellness.

AUSTIN GOES BACK TO NATURE

Medical residency was the most stressful experience of my life. I'd consistently leave the hospital mentally stunned and emotionally drained from providing patient care. I remember sitting on my couch and staring at the wall for far too long, my mind pushed beyond its functional limits. In the winter, I'd ride my bike in the dark to and from work, sometimes missing the sun for days at a time. And this was my daily schedule for up to eighty hours a week.

In my exhausting medical rotations, I was given one day off a week. During this sacred break, I tried to accomplish all the things I had put off in the preceding days. Unfortunately, what should have been my most important task — restoring my mental health — frequently took a back seat to more mundane tasks such as laundry and grocery shopping. Keeping my head above water was a constant struggle. When my day off finally arrived and my basic chores were checked off the list, I found it hard to do much of anything other than sit around and wait for work to start again the next day.

Finally, I hit the breaking point and decided to try something new. Instead of staying home on my day off, I got in my car and drove several hours outside of town into the temperate rain forests of western Oregon and Washington State. It was gloomy, dark, and rainy in the woods. It was amazing. At that time in my life I wasn't aware of the science of nature, but it changed me.

In the forest, I was able to escape the sterile, climate-controlled hospital wards, both physically and mentally.

While trekking through mud and pushing through damp leaves, I was reminded of the beauty of nature and the interconnectedness of living things. I became increasingly thankful for the opportunities in my life and for the health that allowed me to hike through the woods. I also grew increasingly grateful for the opportunity to take care of others.

Nature is the ultimate connector. It's our place of origin and our first home. Our genes developed for millions of years under nature's influences, so it's little wonder that spending time in nature does us good. Distancing ourselves from nature deepens disconnection syndrome, taking us away from well-being and our evolutionary roots. Spending time in nature is one of the easiest things you can do to stay healthy and happy— you just need to step outside. And now we finally have research to prove that our bodies and minds do exceptionally well when prescribed a dose of the outdoors.

Our understanding of the exact mechanisms by which exposure to nature can improve our health may still be in its infancy, but it's important to reflect on what we do know so far. Among other benefits, nature destresses us, lowers inflammation, and increases our empathic behaviors.[3] In essence, it helps rewire the brain for better health, improved focusing abilities, and long-term satisfaction. And nature provides the original antidote to the hectic, stress-addled reality of modern living, reintroducing us to the tangible wonders of the world beyond our screens. This is how nature fights disconnection syndrome. If you're in the middle of the woods or a vast desert, miles away from town, you might not have cell service (this is usually a good thing!). You're also not dealing with the hectic pace and noise of the city. Taking yourself off the grid, even for a short period of time, gives your brain a chance to come up for air. In addition, nature encourages mindfulness, which is a major way to fend off disconnection syndrome. We'll cover mindfulness in detail in chapter 9, but the general gist is that it helps reset our brains, enabling us to look at the world more objectively—activating the prefrontal cortex. And the relationship between nature and mindfulness is reciprocal: nature helps foster mindfulness, and mindfulness allows us to feel more connected to nature.

Nature doesn't just surround us; we *are* nature. Our bodies are microcosms of the vast ecosystem we inhabit. Not only does our cellular makeup, down to our DNA, reflect the perfection of Mother Nature, but we also harbor trillions of beneficial organisms that live inside us and upon us, taking up residence among our own cells. These infinitesimal microbes have been along for the ride for millions of years. We need to recognize the beauty, awesomeness, and health-promoting power inherent in the natural world we inhabit. Let's start by looking at how much has changed.

OUR EVOLUTION IN NATURE

From humble roots on the African savanna, primitive humans migrated across the globe. In each new environment, our ancestors faced challenges requiring adaptation to new temperatures, terrains, and food sources. Throughout our evolution, understanding nature was necessary for survival. We needed to know which plants were edible, which were toxic, and which possessed medicinal qualities. A subtle change in the weather that today would pass unnoticed might well have provided our ancestral humans with lifesaving information. The ebb and flow of the tides and migrations of animals governed our access to nutrition. But we've moved away from nature, literally. In 1900, there were around seven people living in rural environments for every one urbanite. Today, more than one out of every two people—that's half the global population— lives in an urban center, a number expected to grow as the years go by.[4] By 2050, almost 70 percent of us will live in cities.[5] We've found a new home for the modern human, but what is it doing to us?

The truth is, we're not yet sure. This important question has never been studied in detail. That's why the Mayo Clinic has launched a major project called the Well Living Lab.[6] This multiyear research endeavor seeks to understand the impact of the built environment on the health of its occupants. (The phrase "built environment" refers to the artificial, human-made space in which we live, work, and play; it includes everything from high-rises and housing to roads and parks.) The Well Living Lab describes itself as "the first lab exclusively committed to researching the real-world impact of the indoor environment on human health."

What we do know is that children born into the relatively sterile modern world tend to have a higher risk of developing diseases such as asthma, autoimmune disorders, and food allergies than children born in previous centuries. The "hygiene hypothesis" proposes that the uptick in these conditions in Westernized countries may in part be attributable to a lack of exposure to nature and its microbes.[7] It argues that we evolved to benefit from a dose of dirtiness and that the sanitized world we now inhabit confuses our immune systems. Some have suggested we reverse this process by prescribing parasites to children to better develop their immune systems and, ultimately, to help stave off disease! While we're not yet recommending this, the data do make a strong case for a little more nature—a little more dirt—in our lives.

Our move to urban lifestyles has changed our work environments, too, because not many of us are laboring outdoors in fields anymore. Might this come at a cost? A 2016 study looked at whether reintroducing a small amount of nature into an indoor work space could improve mental health.[8] Natural elements in the workplace served as a predictor of overall better health (e.g., lower depression and anxiety) as well as greater job satisfaction. And we're not talking about drastic changes here. These researchers classified potted plants and even photos of nature as "natural elements." It's good to know that just having a picture of a natural scene or having a small plant at work may make a difference. But we're deluding ourselves if we think this is equivalent to the real outdoors. There are no substitutes for fresh air, sunlight, and wild vegetation.

Despite this, Americans spend a remarkable 87 percent of their days indoors and another 6 percent in their cars.[9] Almost the entirety of our interaction with the modern world is taking place within walls of one sort or another—under artificial lighting and in controlled environments. Our main interaction with the outdoors comes through windows, virtual online experiences, and memories. In an illuminating 2018 survey of two thousand Canadians, 87 percent of respondents said they felt happier, healthier, and more productive when they were in nature.[10] However, around 75 percent of them also felt it was simply easier to stay inside. Like domesticated house pets, we've become an indoor species.

This means more than missing out on sun-kissed skin or a breath of fresh air. It results in what journalist and bestselling author Richard Louv calls *nature deficit disorder*.[11] Louv is an advocate for "vitamin N"—*n* for *nature*—and has cofounded an organization that helps connect children, families, and communities to nature. He knows the value and importance of getting back to nature, and you should, too. Let's review some of nature's many contributions to our health, then see exactly why it's such an important tool in fighting disconnection syndrome.

NATURE HEALS

In the 1800s, tuberculosis ran rampant throughout Europe. Despite many attempts at developing an effective treatment, nothing seemed to work. Then the "open air treatment" was created. This protocol emphasized adequate exposure to outside elements, with "fresh air, both by day (out of doors if possible) and by night with wide-open windows,"[12] as described in the *Journal of the Royal Society of Medicine*. It seemed to work far better than anything previously attempted, but nobody knew exactly why. We now believe that some of the benefits conferred may have been the result of sunlight exposure and its critical role in vitamin D production: vitamin D turns on innate immunity to tuberculosis. In the early twentieth century, tuberculosis sanatoriums became common in the United States—this was before the development of antibiotics, so there was nothing else to treat the infection. Arizona's sunshine and dry desert air attracted many people (called lungers) suffering from tuberculosis, rheumatism, asthma, and numerous other diseases. TB camps were formed by pitching tents and building cabins. We knew back then that being outdoors was doing something remarkable for our health, even though we couldn't scientifically explain it. We're just starting to understand exactly why and how nature works this magic.

In 1984, famed biologist Edward O. Wilson described the possible benefits of nature in his biophilia hypothesis. In the 1993 book *The Biophilia Hypothesis,* which was a collection of essays edited by Wilson and social ecologist Stephen Kellert, Kellert proclaims a "human dependence on nature that extends far beyond the simple issues of material and physical sustenance to encompass as well the human craving for aesthetic, intellectual, cognitive and even spiritual meaning and satisfaction."[13] Wilson's biophilia hypothesis suggests that we are innately affiliated with the natural environment in ways that transcend the ideas we usually have about our relationship with nature. We now find ourselves understanding the truth of his theory.

That same year (1984), Dr. Roger Ulrich published a landmark paper in the medical journal *Science* entitled "View Through a Window May Influence Recovery from Surgery."[14] As you might expect, the world of medicine is filled with conversations about the best ways to help patients recover from illness. We've realized that treating an acute issue is only part of the battle and that after surgery, a stroke, a heart attack, or a fight with cancer, the long-term healing process is critical. To this end, we cannot ignore the rapidly expanding field of research showing that nature exposure facilitates recovery from illness and injury.

Dr. Ulrich reviewed the records of postsurgical patients in a Pennsylvania hospital and compared their outcomes to those of patients who were placed in identical rooms—except for a single difference: one set of rooms had windows facing a brick wall, while the other had windows facing a stand of trees. The patients in the rooms facing the trees were discharged earlier and required less pain medication. Their nurses were also one-third less likely to write notes about them that contained such phrases as "upset and crying" and "needs much encouragement." Dr. Ulrich's work went on to influence the way medical centers are designed. Gone are the days of hospitals planned to look like sterile corporate offices: today's designs aim to create a calming environment, with indoor and outdoor gardens, art installations, "living" walls, glazed exteriors that provide light and views, and natural materials such as wood and stone.

Since Dr. Ulrich's revelatory observations, we've seen multiple studies confirming that exposure to nature may significantly improve the healing process. A 2011 paper, for example, looked at 278 patients in a cardiac and pulmonary rehabilitation center in a mountainous village in Norway and compared outcomes in patients with a view of nature to outcomes in patients with a view blocked by buildings.[15] The study found what Dr. Ulrich documented decades earlier:

patients whose windows were blocked by buildings experienced a worsening of physical and mental health compared to patients with an unobstructed view.

Dr. Seong-Hyun Park has been particularly interested in the role of nature in improving recovery from surgery. In one of her studies, she randomly assigned 90 appendectomy patients to identical rooms, save for the fact that some of the rooms contained a plant or flowers.[16] She found that the postoperative group in rooms with plants had significantly lower heart rates and systolic blood pressures compared to the group in rooms without plants. The plant group also needed less pain medication. The participants exposed to plants overwhelmingly rated the greenery as the best thing about their rooms. Their responses to the experience indicated that, compared to the people's experience in the control rooms, the "green" rooms were more "satisfying, relaxing, comfortable, colorful, pleasant smelling, calming, and attractive." Dr. Park has replicated these findings in similar studies since then.

While this may not seem revolutionary on the surface, the fact that a simple potted plant can significantly change hospital outcomes is a big deal. It once again proves our body's gravitational pull toward nature and its healing properties. And though lower blood pressure, lower heart rate, and higher reported relaxation may at first seem unrelated to the brain, they all very much connect to the amygdala and our stress response.

Further research into the benefits of nature on hospital patients shows that plants may not even need to be physically present for patients to benefit from them. In 2012, researchers in Amsterdam set up a hospital waiting room with either real plants, posters of plants, or no plants at all.[17] They were able to show that both the posters of plants and the real plants led to lower levels of stress in patients compared to the plantless waiting room. In another study, conducted by the Mayo Clinic, just a mix of natural sounds and music was able to lower anxiety and pain scores in patients.[18]

Doctors around the world are beginning to take these studies seriously. In 2018 Scottish doctors began to *prescribe* time outdoors. The UK's National Health Service is encouraging doctors to pass out pamphlets written by the Royal Society for the Protection of Birds (RSPB), which offer tips on walks to take and what kind of wildlife to look for. And now there's even a website on which American doctors can print you a prescription for a trip to your favorite park!

SHINRIN-YOKU: FOREST BATHING CALMS, RESTORES, AND CONNECTS US

The Japanese have taken the healing power of nature seriously for a lot longer than average Americans have. They even have a name for the practice of spending time in nature in order to benefit from its healing effects: Shinrin-yoku, which translates as "taking in the forest atmosphere" or "forest bathing."[19] Shinrin-yoku was developed in Japan during the 1980s and has since become a keystone of preventive health care and healing in Japanese medicine. Researchers, primarily in Japan and South Korea, have established a rich body of scientific literature about the health benefits of spending time under the canopy of a living forest. Now their research is helping establish Shinrin-yoku throughout the world. This same research reveals how Shinrin-yoku helps reverse disconnection syndrome.

The idea is simple: if a person visits a natural area and walks in a relaxed way, there are calming, rejuvenating, and restorative benefits to be achieved. We have always known this intuitively (probably because it's built into our instincts). And since the 1980s, science has been catching up with the anecdotal evidence about the healing effects of being in wild and natural areas.

One of the ways that nature seems to exert its effects on our health is through our sense of smell. This may be part of the reason we gravitate toward fresh-smelling trees and flowers and even plant-simulating air fresheners and perfumes. Research has linked the sense of smell to immune function and even mood, cognition, and social behavior.[20] Plant fragrances possess healing qualities in and of themselves. In 1937, the Russian biochemist Boris P. Tokin coined the word *phytoncide* to refer to the substance emitted by plants that helps prevent them from rotting or being eaten by bugs. Phytoncides compose the aroma of the forest, and they are the chemicals that give essential oils their characteristic scents. As it turns out, they may also be quite powerful tools for health, particularly with regard to our immunity.

What's the link between nature scents and immune function? Exposure to nature has been shown to increase our immune-cell populations. In one trial, researchers measured the blood and urine of female nurses during a typical workday, then again after they spent three days and two nights in a forest.[21] The researchers found a significant increase in the nurses' blood levels of "natural killer" cells and a significant decrease in their urine levels of adrenaline and noradrenaline, two of the major chemicals of the sympathetic nervous system and the stress response. Natural killer cells, sometimes abbreviated as NKs, are crucial to the body's ability to fight off viruses and tumors. These results indicate that the nurses got a boost to their immune systems and a lowered level of sympathetic nervous system activation after their forest trip. Researchers conducted a similar trial with male volunteers, finding that one day in nature led to significant increases in blood NK cells as well as a drop in urine levels of adrenaline.[22] In both studies, the researchers believe these effects may be attributable to the phytoncides in the forest. They also link phytoncides to lower levels of stress, which may have then led to improved immune function. Just as important as the immune-boosting effect, however, is the destressing effect that nature had in these trials. Remember, chronic stress takes the prefrontal cortex offline, so by lowering our stress hormones, nature is giving us a great tool in maintaining higher-level thinking.

Part of the allure of essential oils (phytoncides) is the relaxation we feel upon inhaling them (there's a reason they're popular in spas). So it's no surprise that yet another study looking at the effects of inhaling the scent of cedarwood oil (called cedrol) found that it led to increased parasympathetic activity, which is generally associated with a relaxed state.[23] Parasympathetic activity was also increased in a study that examined the effect of smelling oil from the cypress plant.[24] It's worth noting that the relaxation-associated parasympathetic system counterbalances the stress-related sympathetic system (fight or flight). A healthy balance of these two systems is important. But what part of the brain keeps us stuck in sympathetic mode? You guessed it: the amygdala.

Studies conducted since 2010 on the effects of aroma on human brain function have been astonishing. They show that the mere sniff of a certain scent can shift brain waves and activity from those associated with disease and cognitive decline to those linked with health and wellness. How is this possible? Turns out that fragrance compounds are able to cross the blood-brain barrier and interact with receptors in the central nervous system. The blood-brain barrier is a biological gate between the blood and the brain, keeping potentially harmful substances from damaging the central nervous system. A 2016 paper reviewing several studies states: "The olfactory stimulation of fragrances produces immediate changes in physiological parameters such as blood pressure, muscle tension, pupil dilation, skin temperature, pulse rate, and brain activity."[25] The paper describes these connections in detail, explaining the ways in which various scents, from bunches of fresh lavender and chamomile to incense and essential oils, affect diverse parts of the brain. The researchers conclude that "fragrances directly and/or indirectly affect the psychological and physiological conditions of humans" and that "fragrances significantly modulate the activities of different brain waves and are responsible for various states of the brain." That should give us all something to think about the next time we smell flowers or a wonderful perfume.

And certainly the health benefits of nature exposure appear to be far more widespread than just what we gain through our noses. Forest-bathing research is, as it were, blossoming. More of the health-boosting effects of this practice are being discovered every year. At this point the scientifically studied benefits include:

- boosted immune-system functioning, with an increase in the count and activity of the body's natural killer cells;

- reduced blood pressure;
- heightened coping abilities for stress and less stress in general;
- improved mood;
- increased mindfulness;
- increased ability to focus, even in children with ADHD;
- accelerated recovery from surgery or illness;
- increased energy; and
- improved sleep.

> "Thousands of tired, nerve-shaken, over-civilized people are beginning to find out that going to the mountains is going home. Wilderness is a necessity."
>
> — John Muir

Though it may seem intuitive, it's important to review the ways in which the outdoors can significantly affect our moods. As we wrote in chapter 1, rates of depression and suicide have gone up significantly in our lifetimes. But our current treatments for depression leave much to be desired. In fact, the only evidence-based options currently prescribed by doctors are drugs and cognitive behavioral therapy (CBT)—psychotherapy designed to change negative thoughts and behaviors. But even the benefits of CBT may be enhanced by nature. One particularly fascinating study looked at whether undergoing CBT outdoors would increase the potency of the technique.[26] In the study, one group received CBT in a hospital setting while the other group was given the same treatment in a forest. The study found that the forest group experienced a 61 percent decrease in depression symptoms as measured by established depression scales, whereas the hospital group experienced only a 21 percent decrease.

Another study looked at the connection between the amount of time people spend in green space and the risk of developing depression.[27] No surprise: it found a significantly lower risk of depression in those who spend five hours or more per week in nature, concluding that "nearby nature offers huge potential as an easily accessible and cost-effective approach to illness prevention."

Let's flip the coin to the other side of this conversation: What does science say about nature increasing happiness (as opposed to the decreasing risk of depression)? In 2014, a meta-analysis examined whether nature was linked to happiness. The study reviewed trials that included around 8,500 individuals and found that "those who are more connected to nature tended to experience more positive affect, vitality, and life satisfaction compared to those less connected to nature."[28] A rather modern technique for studying the role of nature on our happiness is the use of GPS location services. In one nifty study, researchers asked twenty thousand participants about their moods at random intervals—and compared this information to where they were located.[29] Were they in a park or building? The researchers amassed around one million responses, showing that people were significantly happier when their GPS coordinates were near green or natural habitats as opposed to urban environments.

> "One touch of nature makes the whole world kin."
> — William Shakespeare

One of the ways nature is believed to exert its healthful effects is by combating stress. Of course this makes a lot of sense. The words *relaxation* and *nature* go together for a reason. As we mentioned earlier, nature activates the relaxation-promoting parasympathetic nervous system, dampening the stress-promoting sympathetic nervous system. It also has been shown to lower cortisol levels. So if nature helps us manage chronic stress, it may very well be handing us back the reins for better self-control, more thoughtful decisions, and improved regulation of our emotions and impulsivity— because we know that chronic stress damages the prefrontal cortex and strengthens the amygdala. Put simply, nature allows us to regain control of our brains and helps relieve disconnection syndrome.

> "For all Nature is doing her best each moment to make us well. She exists for no other end. Do not resist her."
>
> — Henry David Thoreau

Nature's mood-boosting power owes some credit to the sun. When those rays hit your skin, you make vitamin D, a hormone that's not only critical to a wide variety of biological processes but is also directly tied to the brain's ability to synthesize serotonin. This was well described by Dr. Rhonda Patrick, a scientist who studies aging and disease prevention.[30] She postulates that vitamin D deficiency, a condition that is prevalent among Americans, may contribute to depression. Most commonly prescribed medications designed to improve mood purportedly work by increasing available serotonin. But this new research proposes that simply increasing vitamin D levels, either by getting out in the sunshine or by taking a vitamin D supplement, may well improve mood, likely by boosting serotonin.

Here is where some of the science has become breathtaking: nature exposure may change our behavior for the better. And it may do this by inducing *awe,* or wonder. In a riveting series of studies, Dr. Paul Piff and his colleagues at the University of California at Irvine looked at the impact of nature exposure and the role of awe in changing our behavioral tendencies. Dr. Piff describes awe as "an emotional response to perceptually vast stimuli that transcend current frames of reference."[31] In their research, his team showed that inducing awe led to increased ethical decision making, generosity, and prosocial values. They then demonstrated that triggering awe through exposure to a group of tall trees led to "enhanced prosocial behavior and decreased entitlement." Awe seems uniquely powerful. There's a feeling of time almost standing still when you witness something awe-inspiring, especially upon first experiencing it. Think of a moment when you stood before a gushing waterfall or watched a rainbow grow stronger in its coloring. Didn't it make you feel calm and connected rather than anxious and disconnected?

In 2012 researchers proved that this feeling is measurable, showing that compared to other emotions, a sense of awe made participants feel they had more time available.[32] What's more, in this same group of experiments, those who experienced awe were more willing to volunteer and "more strongly preferred experiences over material products." The researchers concluded that "experiences of awe bring people into the present moment…[making] life feel more satisfying than it would otherwise."

It's impressive and motivating to think that when we see awe-inspiring nature, we experience a significant and positive effect on the way we interact with others. The awe that comes from nature reminds us of our relatively insignificant place in the universe, allowing us to focus on others without disproportionately overvaluing our self-worth. Awe also displaces some of the materialistic desires that lead us down the rabbit hole of unhappiness and constant comparison. These potent benefits are important in a world that fosters narcissism and materialism. Awe can change our outlook for the better and facilitate empathic behaviors. It simply makes us better people, resistant to disconnection syndrome.

In another series of experiments conducted by Dr. Piff, his group looked at the ways in which exposure to beauty in nature changed people's perspectives.[33] The researchers found that "exposure to more beautiful images of nature (versus less beautiful images of nature) led participants to be more generous and trusting" and that "exposure to more beautiful (versus less beautiful) plants in the laboratory room led participants to exhibit increased helping behavior." This research further highlights the fact that exposure to nature can create a measurable prosocial benefit. We're literally the best versions of ourselves when we enjoy the sunset or take a hike (ideally with a friend).

Where does empathy come in? Scientists have studied this in two different ways, but both show the power of nature to increase empathic behavior. In one set of experiments, participants were exposed to scenery from either an urban or a natural landscape, then had their brains imaged with fMRI to see which parts were more active.[34] Not surprisingly, the amygdala lit up more in the participants who viewed the urban scenery compared to the participants shown a natural landscape. As for the other experiment, what do you think happens when you put a preteen in the woods without any screen-based media for five days? This question was answered in 2014, when fifty-one preteens "spent five days at an overnight nature camp where television, computers, and mobile phones were not allowed."[35] Back in town, fifty-four kids of a similar age continued their use of smartphones, tablets, TV, computers, and all other screens as usual. Before and after the five-day period, both groups of kids were shown photos and videos of people and asked to determine their emotional states. This was a way of gauging how well the kids could perceive the emotions of others. The findings were telling. The preteens who spent five days cut off from digital media were significantly better at recognizing emotional cues in others—an important skill for successful interpersonal connection and the expression of empathy. A few days in nature, away from screens, made all the difference.

If we know that the ability to express empathy appears to require a functional prefrontal cortex, and if nature appears to improve empathy, then we shouldn't be surprised to find further links between a strong prefrontal cortex and connection to nature. In fact, a 2019 paper, published in the journal *Scientific Reports*, showed that higher activation in the prefrontal cortex was associated with "higher frequency of everyday pro-environmental behavior."[36] It seems the link between the prefrontal cortex and nature is bidirectional. They support each other.

It's important to note that nature has anti-inflammatory effects, too, which in turn may help keep the prefrontal cortex healthy and engaged. Multiple studies have confirmed this finding. For example, a 2012 trial measured the differences in blood markers of stress and inflammation among college men sent into either the woods or a city.[37] In the lab work done before the experiment, there were no significant differences in the levels of stress markers and inflammation between the two groups of men. But after two nights in the woods or the city, it was a different story. In the woods group, levels of the inflammatory markers TNF alpha and interleukin 6 were significantly reduced compared to the city group. The levels of endothelin 1, a marker of inflammation in vascular diseases, was also lower in the woods group, as were levels of the stress hormone cortisol, which as you'll recall is implicated in severing the connection between the prefrontal cortex and the amygdala.

If you're still on the fence, or if you feel your need to be productive outweighs the need to spend time outside, there's something else to add. Nature (and the associated break from digital ties) may give you a substantial cognitive boost. A 2012 study tested fifty-six men and women in creative problem solving before and after a four-day nature hike.[38] The researchers found that "four days of immersion in nature, and the corresponding disconnection from multimedia and technology, increases performance [on problem-solving tasks that require creativity] by a full 50%." Regardless of whether you like to hike, that's nothing to sneeze at.

Nature's positive effect on our ability to focus and concentrate has long been documented. There's even something called attention restoration theory (ART), which psychologists Stephen and Rachel Kaplan developed in the late 1980s and early 1990s, a period characterized by rapid technological advancement and ever-increasing indoor activity and concerns about nature deficit. ART hypothesizes that nature, in addition to honing our ability to focus and concentrate, helps renew our attention after we exert mental energy—for example, after we spend sleepless nights working tirelessly on a project or an assignment. Nature restores our brains by reinforcing the connections that allow us to focus and concentrate in the first place: those of the prefrontal cortex.

In the bigger picture, scientists have been examining the way nature affects our entire life span and have reached some striking conclusions. A colossal 2008 study in *The Lancet* looked at forty million English people and classified them by how "green" their living environments were—i.e., how much green space there was within a few kilometers of their homes. Green space was defined as "open, undeveloped land with natural vegetation" and included parks, forests, woodlands, and playing fields.[39] The researchers found that people living in the greenest areas had the lowest rates of dying from circulatory diseases and lived longer than those whose environments were less green. In another large study, this one conducted in 2017 and involving 1.7 million Canadians, the risk of dying prematurely was around 10 percent lower in people who lived with a lot of greenery around their residences.[40] And yet another big 2017 study analyzed 4.2 million Swiss people and showed the same associations: residential greenery lowered the risk of dying prematurely, even when controlled for pollution and other harmful environmental exposures.[41] An earlier large review of available studies concluded the same thing in 2015.[42]

The one key takeaway from all these studies is that nature heals and connects. And it does so through an array of mechanisms that are chemical (for example, by decreasing stress hormones and inflammation) and neurological (for example, by improving attention and memory function). Nature ultimately rewires the brain for peaceful well-being and supports the body's overall physiology. It can positively interact with our immune systems and physically alter brain waves, changing activity across the brain to promote prosocial, altruistic behavior as opposed to the materialistic and self-centered tendencies that define disconnection syndrome. It is clear that we need nature to thrive. And its benefits are within our grasp today.

During the program, we'll suggest that you enjoy nature by combining it with another Brain Wash activity, such as meditating. You can sit in solitude in nature or take it in with a friend. You can exercise in nature. Eat outdoors. And so on...

In a world that's constantly threatening to keep us from becoming the compassionate, empathic, forward-thinking beings we aspire to be, how wonderful it is to know that simply exposing ourselves to nature can help set things right. Tomorrow, see if you can wake up to natural sunlight: open your windows if weather permits. Buy a plant for your office. Try an essential oil. And plan to be in nature for at least thirty minutes a week—minimum! This means scheduling walks in the park or hikes in local mountains (bonus: with a friend or two). Aim to exercise outdoors when you can. Consider an ecotour for your next vacation. Nature is a main ingredient in your brain wash, and when the health benefits of nature are so easy to realize, the "green pill" should be a standard prescription for all of us.

CHAPTER 7

Clear the Table

Food for Thought

The food you eat can be either the safest and most powerful form of medicine or the slowest form of poison.

—Ann Wigmore

In the first part of the twentieth century, an unofficial experiment of unprecedented scale and significance quietly began in the United States. Chemically altered food substitutes were fed to millions of people. These nutrient-depleted meals were deployed across the nation, replacing real foods with bioengineered surrogates. Billions of dollars were spent on the experiment, allowing food producers to make these products incredibly addictive and readily available. Marketers used the latest science to take advantage of the human brain. Famous people from the world of sports and entertainment were hired to promote these synthetic meals as if they could enhance everyone's life (and looks). This massive experiment had no restrictions on age, race, or gender. The government helped pay for it. The results of this manipulation of the American diet have been nothing short of catastrophic.

In the decades since this ongoing experiment commenced, the consequences have become painfully obvious. Many of those who participated developed obesity, diabetes, cardiovascular disease, cancer, and dementia. Their bodies and brains started to fail them. The experimenters denied responsibility, placing the blame on the people who had eaten their toxic food products. And the enormous experiment continues unchecked. Americans take part with every mouthful of processed, engineered food they consume. And they don't come close to looking like the celebrities who peddle these foods daily. Not only are the majority of us overweight or obese, we also suffer from chronic, preventable illnesses as a result of our food choices. It's exactly as Dr. Robert Lustig, a pediatric endocrinologist, said in a 2017 paper: "Processed food is an experiment that failed."[1]

A large-scale study published in the *Journal of the American Medical Association* in 2019 reached a sweeping conclusion: increased consumption of processed food is associated with a 14 percent increase in risk for "all-cause mortality."[2] Another study released in 2019, published in *The Lancet* and equally jaw-dropping, stated that globally, one in five deaths in 2017 was associated with poor diet.[3] These statistics are a flagrant indication of widespread disconnection syndrome. When we choose to eat poorly, we suffer serious consequences. We are disconnected from the foods that nourish our brains and bodies.

The move away from real food does more than cause diseases such as diabetes and heart failure. As we began to explain in chapter 1, modern, ultraprocessed food is a form of biological warfare, taking over your brain's decision making and emotional regulation. It activates addictive brain networks, creating some of the most potent pathways to disease that exist. We often talk about the role of food as medicine, but we must address the terrifying potential of our typical diet to reshape our thoughts, actions, and overall brain makeup.

Food science has never been more complicated than it is today. If you could get deep inside the manufacturing plants of any of the largest food and beverage companies, you'd be shocked to see what they do. And yes, some of the rooms do resemble scientific laboratories, where food technologists wear white lab coats and sport eye goggles. Before modern food processing methods, our meals were grown, raised, or foraged. Today, food labels feature an astonishing number of substances engineered in a chemistry lab. You probably cannot pronounce, for example, tetrasodium pyrophosphate, acetylated monoglycerides, and thiamine mononitrate. It's much easier to say "chicken nuggets," "croissants," and "cream-filled cookies."

The American government has finally retreated from its position endorsing a low-fat, high-carbohydrate diet. But by financially contributing to the production of corn (and other agricultural products, such as wheat and soy, that are often converted into refined, highly processed foods), it indirectly continues to subsidize the addition of high-fructose corn syrup in everything from meat to ketchup. This means American taxpayers are paying to have sugar added to their foods (and paying yet again for the diseases that excess sugar will inevitably cause). These facts alone should give us pause when we consider whether the government's dietary recommendations really have our best interests at heart.

Food additives are a massive industry. According to the Food and Drug Administration (FDA), a food additive is "any substance the intended use of which results or may reasonably be expected to result (directly or indirectly) in its becoming a component or otherwise affecting the characteristics of any food."[4] The FDA's website outlines the various ways that food additives such as colored dyes are incorporated into our diet, stating that "color additives are now recognized as an important part of practically all processed foods we eat."[5] Their article summary concludes with the reassurance that "consumers should feel safe about the foods they eat."

What a quaint statement. The government tells us that what we're eating is safe. Unfortunately, the data show otherwise. The foods we eat are not necessarily "safe," at least not from the perspective of what the standard American diet can do to the body in the long term. We no longer doubt that this standard diet is a central cause of diseases such as diabetes, stroke, heart disease, high blood pressure, cancer, and dementia, including Alzheimer's disease. We also know these diseases are among the top causes of death in the United States.

The FDA states that "additives perform a variety of useful functions in foods that consumers often take for granted."[6] Shelf life and freshness are useful, but sweetness? In 2016, researchers at the University of North Carolina sought to find out how common added sweeteners are in food products.[7] They looked at 1.2 million foods sold in the United States and found that an astonishing 68 percent had added sweeteners. In 2019, researchers at Harvard's T. H. Chan School of Public Health published a large-scale study showing that people who drink two or more servings of sugar-sweetened drinks a day have a 31 percent higher risk of dying early from cardiovascular disease than do those who indulge less frequently.[8] The increased risk was particularly strong among women. Diet drinks aren't a viable alternative, either. In the same study, women who drank four or more artificially sweetened drinks a day had an increased risk of early death, too.

Food companies are adding an addictive, toxic substance to most foods. We're hooked. And yet we have a habit of blaming only the consumers when they are unable to stop themselves from eating and drinking these products. The first step to dietary change requires understanding what you're actually eating, how you're being manipulated to eat the wrong things, and how those dietary choices are affecting your brain—preventing you from using your prefrontal cortex to make good dietary decisions! Let's start with what precipitated our current food crisis: the agricultural revolution.

HISTORY'S BIGGEST FOOD FRAUD

The development of agriculture—the domestication of plants and animals—occurred around twelve thousand years ago and unfolded almost simultaneously in many areas around the world, including Europe, Africa, South America, and Asia. The swing toward agriculture-based subsistence and away from the hunter-gatherer lifestyle is partially responsible for a marked increase in population growth. But while we increased in number, our diets suffered. As we learned to farm and grow crops, we began to eat more calories than we needed, and the human diet suddenly shifted to one that focused on far fewer types of foods. This reduction in diversity may well constitute the most dramatic dietary shift in human history. With the lack of diversity came a lack of nutrients. And as our dietary choices became narrower, we grew wider.

Dr. Amanda Mummert is a research scientist at IBM Watson Health who studies the history of human health and cultural factors in disease processes. According to her, "empirical studies of societies shifting subsistence from foraging to primary food production have found evidence for deteriorating health from an increase in infectious and dental disease and a rise in nutritional deficiencies."[9] Let's put that into plain language:

Development of agriculture → decreased food diversity → more disease

Jared Diamond is one of the world's leading historians and geographers. He is also a Pulitzer Prize–winning author who has written extensively about the impact of agriculture on human health. He calls agriculture "the worst mistake in the history of the human race."[10] He notes that hunter-gatherers had a highly variable diet in contrast to early farmers, who received most of their sustenance from only a few carbohydrate-based crops. Diamond also points out that the trade fostered by the agricultural revolution may have led to the spread of parasites and infectious diseases. He goes as far as saying that the adoption of agriculture "was in many ways a catastrophe from which we have never recovered."[11] Historian Yuval Noah Harari echoed this sentiment in his bestselling book *Sapiens:* "The Agricultural Revolution certainly enlarged the sum total of food at the disposal of humankind, but the extra food did not translate into a better diet or more leisure... The Agricultural Revolution was history's biggest fraud."[12]

CARBS SPEAK ANOTHER LANGUAGE

We've long known that food is information. The foods we consume send signals from our environment to our life code, our DNA. Every bit of food we consume changes the expression of our genes, meaning the way our DNA is turned into messages and building blocks for our bodies. Think about that fact alone: you have the ability to alter, for better or worse, the activity of your DNA! We call this alteration, brought about by the effects of extrinsic influences, *epigenetics*. And, as it turns out, more than 90 percent of the genetic switches in our DNA that are associated with longevity are significantly influenced by our lifestyle choices, including the foods we eat.[13] For example, a diet rich in refined carbohydrates decreases the activity of the gene that makes brain-protective BDNF.[14] However, when we eat healthful fats and proteins (which was common among our preagricultural ancestors), the activity of the gene pathway increases the production of BDNF.

It makes sense that our DNA works best with an ancient diet. For more than 99 percent of the time we have existed on this planet, we have eaten a diet much lower in refined carbohydrates, higher in healthful fat and fiber, and, equally important, much more diverse than our diets are now. In fact our modern-day Western diet works against our DNA's ability to protect health and longevity. And we experience the consequences of this mismatch every day.

> The importance of food goes well beyond its nutrient content. Moment to moment, our food choices allow each of us to control our gene expression.

Foods can enhance or reduce inflammation. Foods can enhance or reduce our bodies' ability to detoxify and create important antioxidants. And because our food choices influence the structure and functioning of our brains, they can either help us remain grounded or cause us to become fearful, threatened, and impulsive. Now, this is where science is gaining traction and getting exciting. Food may be the most powerful tool for changing how we behave and think.

While there are healthful foods that can result from modern farming, in general Big Agriculture produces a lot of processed foods (the term *Big Ag* is often used to refer to farming by large corporations — not your local mom-and-pop farmer). The economics of this business have moved our country toward a diet rich in inflammatory, disease-inducing refined carbohydrates, a clear and present danger to our ability to access and make use of higher-order thinking.

You've probably heard that a diet high in refined carbs paves the way for blood sugar elevation (and if you're diabetic, then you definitely know this to be true from your own experience). High blood sugar is associated not only with virtually every chronic degenerative condition there is but also, even when it's just mildly elevated, with a well-documented increased risk of brain shrinkage and even dementia. As outlined in a report in the *Journal of Alzheimer's Disease,* having blood sugar levels above the normal range was associated with a dramatically increased risk of developing dementia![15] Why does elevated blood sugar threaten the brain? In a word: inflammation.

Big Ag + Big Food = Big Problem. A large number of calories now come from refined carbohydrates, especially sugar. And when it comes to our food budget, we've nearly doubled the share we spend on processed foods and sweets (from 11.6 percent to 22.9 percent in thirty years).[16] According to researchers at Tufts University, "prescribing" fruits and vegetables would save $100 billion in medical costs in the United States alone.[17]

THE MANIPULATION BEGINS EARLY

Think back to childhood. Can you remember your favorite cereal? Can you recall the TV ad for it or the box it came in — perhaps even the cartoon character affiliated with that brand? Your memories of that food are likely pleasant, invoking nostalgia. You have been conditioned to associate food with positive emotion. Research shows that this positive feeling creates a bias toward the product that lingers into adulthood. That same bias is being instilled in our children through advertising. But why does it matter?

The food-advertising industry wants us to make unhealthful choices. It has focused its efforts on the easiest and most vulnerable targets—children. This isn't to say that adults are immune. But the cycle of life-long consumption of junk food begins with marketing these toxic products to the youngest generation. From multiple studies around the world, we see that advertisements for children's food focus on unhealthful fare such as crackers, chips, juice boxes, sugary snacks, and ultraprocessed fast foods.

The goal is clear. It's a multifaceted, multibillion-dollar marketing program designed to capture the minds of our children and turn our youngest Americans into lifelong customers. Strategies to achieve this seem to respect no boundaries. Advertisements for food products find their way into school curricula when companies sponsor lesson plans. Fast-food restaurants give away food and beverages to high-achieving students, fostering the association of academic success with junk food in young minds. And TV commercials for unhealthful foods are in heavy rotation. The scariest part? The foods themselves may change the development of children's brains.

This is not only an American problem. Worldwide studies are finally calling for improved regulation of these product pitches. One Canadian study found that

Canadians were "failing to protect children from... [the] marketing [of foods] high in fat, sugar, and sodium on television,"[18] and a Mexican study found that "the majority of foods and beverages advertised on Mexican TV do not comply with any nutritional quality standards, and thus should not be marketed to children."[19] A study reviewing TV commercials in Spain found that "over half the commercials were for less healthy products."[20] Most succinctly, a recent Iranian study of TV ads for children's food concludes, "TV food commercials do not encourage healthy eating."[21]

The chief issue with these ads is that they promote an increase in caloric intake, especially from low-quality foods and drinks. In a 2009 study, young children exposed to TV food ads consumed 45 percent more food in general,[22] and a more recent meta-analysis confirms that children who are exposed to ads "eat significantly more than those who are not."[23] In 2019, the media were buzzing around a paper written by researchers at Dartmouth College that showed that TV ads for high-sugar breakfast cereals directed at children increased the amount of cereal children ate. Of course, that's the point of the advertising, but is it right to manipulate preschoolers and get them hooked on these harmful products? The study's authors state, "Findings indicate child-directed advertising influences begin earlier and last longer than previously demonstrated, highlighting limitations of current industry guidelines regarding the marketing of high-sugar foods to children under age 6 years."[24]

Our children are being swayed to favor addictive, unhealthful food choices. The consequences for their brains and bodies will last a lifetime. This is how disconnection syndrome takes root.

As this population grows older, it becomes increasingly difficult for them to avoid the results of poor food choices. Obesity could be a life sentence for them. And as it relates to the brain, obesity is strongly associated with increased impulsivity and chronic inflammation. We get addicted young and stay sick for life.

Corporations do their best to connect food with emotions such as happiness and activities such as recreation and sex to influence our buying patterns. One study, for example, conducted by researchers from New York University, Harvard, the University of Pennsylvania, Duke University, and the University of Cincinnati, found that 76 percent of the foods advertised during sporting events were unhealthful.[25] Dr. Marie Bragg, the lead author of this study, also investigated food and beverage endorsements made by famous athletes. She and her team found that sports celebrities tend to overwhelmingly recommend poor dietary choices: a full 79 percent of the foods they endorse qualify as energy-dense and nutrient-poor. Even worse, almost all the calories in the beverages they hawk come directly from added sugar. And these celebrity athletes are role models for our youth. Dr. Bragg's paper even drew parallels between the food industry's sponsorship of athletes and the tactics used by the tobacco industry in years gone by.

THE WRONG REWARDS

It's important to understand that the neuroscience of addiction involves activation of specific pathways in the brain. We wrote about this in chapter 3, explaining that dopamine surges keep us coming back for more. There are two general ways food affects our thoughts and decisions: (1) food affects inflammation pathways that reach the brain and change its wiring, and (2) food affects addiction circuitry. These two processes go hand in hand.

We're now learning that our craving for sugar, for example, doesn't just start in the brain. In fact, there appears to be a link between inflammatory excess abdominal (visceral) fat and the activation of our dopamine-based reward system.[26] Our belly fat seems to have its own agenda—keeping us fat!

"We don't get fat because we overeat; we overeat because we're getting fat."
—Gary Taubes, *Why We Get Fat: And What to Do About It*

Poor dietary choices lead to increased abdominal fat, creating inflammation and making us impulsive and more likely to eat the foods that pack on the pounds. This might help explain the high levels of impulsive behavior documented in obese people.[27] Inflammation associated with obesity has also predicted worse executive function in both adolescents and adults.[28] Just how powerful is the influence of food on our addictive circuits? A 2013 study conducted at the University of Southern California revealed that the mere sight of high-calorie, pro-inflammatory foods can promote overeating by stimulating brain reward pathways and appetite.[29] Reward circuits lit up when the women who participated in the study saw the unhealthful options. And it's the activation of these reward circuits that make it so hard to stop. What made this particular study unique is that the researchers made a connection between volume of belly fat and how strongly the reward pathways in the brain fired. Most concerning, they found that the wider the waist circumference, the stronger the activation in the addiction circuits of the brain. **Our fat cells are accomplices in keeping us hooked, ultimately blocking us from connecting to our prefrontal cortices and thus preventing us from making good dietary decisions.**

One of the ways scientists study abdominal obesity is by measuring the waist-to-hip ratio (WHR). A high WHR generally indicates the presence of a high level of abdominal fat. In 2012, researchers indicated that women with a high WHR exhibited less empathy than those with a low WHR, but by contrast, "women with low WHRs [excelled] at identifying emotional states of other people."[30] Make no mistake: fat around your middle could be shaping your thoughts and decision making for the worse. Our goal is to break this vicious cycle.

New research shows exactly how our unhealthful intake of refined carbohydrates can change our preferences. One trial looked at the difference between meals high and low in refined carbs and found that people who ate high-carbohydrate meals had significantly more activation of the nucleus accumbens, a core component of the reward pathway.[31] Persistent consumption of refined carbs may then lead the brain to see these foods as rewards, reinforcing this unhealthful link. As these connections grow stronger, it becomes harder to say no to that sugary, starchy treat.

Could our glaring rates of obesity be the result of an overactivation of the reward system and an underactivation of the prefrontal cortex, leading to an impaired ability to say no to unhealthful foods? In an illuminating 2018 study, an international team of researchers developed a framework for understanding problematic food consumption.[32] The researchers argued that an overactive reward system and an underactive control system could be two of the major players that determine whether we eat healthful or unhealthful foods. They conclude, "This loss of control over food consumption can explain, at least in part, the development of excess weight and contribute to the obesity epidemic."

Other published research further adds to the picture by examining a link between an active amygdala and the risk of developing type 2 diabetes.[33] We know that type 2 diabetes is primarily caused by lifestyle choices, especially a diet high in sugar and refined carbs. We also know that diabetes is tightly linked to inflammation. In this study, researchers showed that activation of the amygdala was elevated when inflammation was high. More important, they demonstrated—for the first time—that people who had the most active amygdalas were by far the most likely to develop type 2 diabetes, regardless of whether they were obese.

We've seen the effects of a poor diet on the brain. What about the effects of a healthful diet? A study of 672 adults (with an average age of 79.8) compared the participants' dietary habits with the thickness of their brain cortices.[34] It found that those adults who consumed Mediterranean-style diets—low in refined carbohydrates and red meat and high in healthful fats—had thicker cortices, including a thicker prefrontal cortex. In other words, your food could determine how well you think.

Speaking of healthful fats, we should point out that omega-3 fatty acids are dietary darlings for two big reasons. One, they are among the most powerful anti-inflammatories we consume. And two, they have been shown to have an impact on the brain's high-level thinking. A 2013 study demonstrated that high blood levels of omega-3s were specifically linked to the preservation of executive function as people age,[35] while another trial found that the omega-3 fatty acid EPA might provide the valuable effect of improving oxygenation in the prefrontal cortex.[36] During the ten-day Brain Wash, you'll be consuming lots of these healthful fats.

FOOD SPEAKS TO MORE THAN JUST YOU

We've all heard that women who are pregnant need to watch what they eat because they are "eating for two." But when you consider that our food choices affect our resident microbes, each and every one of us is "eating for trillions." Not only does food supply nutrients to our cells, it also nourishes our trillions of gut bacteria, changing their genetic expression as well. Why is this significant? Let's take a brief detour to examine this important fact.

Gut bacteria are key to our survival. Collectively, our microbial comrades are referred to as our microbiome, and they play a role in many physiological functions: they manufacture neurotransmitters and vitamins that we couldn't otherwise produce, promote normal gastrointestinal function, provide protection from infection, regulate metabolism and the absorption of food, and help control blood sugar balance. They even affect whether we are overweight or lean, hungry or satiated. Because the health of the microbiome factors into immune-system function and inflammation levels, those microbes may ultimately factor into the risk for illnesses as varied as depression, obesity, bowel disorders, diabetes, multiple sclerosis, asthma, autism, Alzheimer's disease, Parkinson's disease, and even cancer. They also help control gut permeability—the integrity of your intestinal wall, which acts as a gatekeeper of sorts. A break in the intestinal wall allows food toxins and pathogens to pass into the bloodstream, triggering an aggressive and often prolonged immune response. This breach affects not only the gut but also other organs and tissues, including the skeletal system, the skin, the kidneys, the pancreas, the liver, and the brain.

The book *Brain Maker* covered the science of the microbiome in depth, and we encourage you to read it to learn more.[37] The Brain Wash program is designed to cultivate a healthy microbiome, which will help optimize brain function. The risk factors for an unhealthy intestinal microbiome are within your control. They include diets high in refined carbohydrates, sugar, artificial sweeteners, lack of exercise, stress, and even not getting enough restorative sleep. Conversely, there's a lot you can do to nourish the health of your microbiome, including eating probiotic-rich fermented foods such as kimchi and cultured yogurt and adding prebiotic-rich foods to your plate. Prebiotics are like fertilizer for your microbes, helping them grow and reproduce. They can be found in common foods such as garlic, onions, leeks, and asparagus. You can also support your gut bugs by avoiding genetically modified organisms (GMO) and eating organic food whenever possible. In animal studies, the herbicides used on GMO crops have been shown to negatively alter the microbiome.

> Our food has been modified in part by the pesticides, herbicides, hormones, and antibiotics we use. Eating organic food, though more expensive than conventionally grown food, is a way of regaining control of the chemical messages that enter your body. When it comes to food expenditures, you either pay more for healthful food now or spend a lot more later to treat the diseases that result.

HOW FOOD GETS YOU DOWN

What is the link between food and depression? Again, we turn to the role of inflammation. When you think of depression, chemical imbalances probably come to mind. The general understanding is still that depression is caused by chemical imbalances in the brain. But this simple explanation is falling out of favor in the scientific literature. Depression is a complex mental illness. Multiple factors are at play. For example, research has shown that depression is an inflammatory disorder. The same inflammatory markers we see elevated in heart disease are also elevated in people suffering from depression. We've only just begun to understand the depths of this connection, thanks to better technology and longitudinal study. High levels of inflammation are associated with a dramatic increase in the risk of developing depression. And the higher the levels of inflammatory markers—notably, C-reactive protein—the worse the depression.[38] A 2013 meta-analysis of this hypothesis reaffirmed the relationship between inflammation and depression.[39] In fact, several studies were under way in 2019 to determine whether depression can be treated with anti-inflammatory medications. This places depression in the same category as other inflammatory disorders such as diabetes, multiple sclerosis, Alzheimer's disease, and obesity. While these ailments are distinct, they share a common denominator: rampant inflammation.

Anything that can cause chronic, systemic inflammation will increase one's risk for developing depression as well as fuel the condition if it already exists. And you know where we're going with this: sugar. An increasingly clear link is being documented between sugar and depression. A 2002 study found "a highly significant correlation between sugar consumption and the annual rate of depression."[40] A 2018 study of more than fifteen thousand adults showed that high sugar consumption was associated with a 35 percent increase in the risk of developing depression.[41] It's not only the sugar, though. Refined carbohydrates are the culprits, too. A 2015 study uncovered an increased risk of depression in postmenopausal women who ate a diet high in rapidly digested, refined carbohydrates.[42] On the opposite end of the spectrum, the Mediterranean diet—low in carbohydrates and rich in olive oil, nuts, and seeds—was correlated with a more than 30 percent *reduced* risk of depression, according to a 2018 review of several large studies.[43]

Your gut bugs also play a role in your mood and emotional stability. This is an active and fascinating area of research, a large volume of which has demonstrated a dynamic communication highway between the brain and the digestive system. Through this two-way connection, the brain receives information about what's going on in your intestines and sends information back to your gut to ensure optimal functioning. All this transmission back and forth helps you control your eating behavior and digestion. The gut also sends out hormonal signals that trigger feelings of fullness, hunger, and even pain from intestinal inflammation.

We doctors see this clearly in diseases that target the intestines. Conditions such as uncontrolled celiac disease, irritable bowel syndrome, and inflammatory bowel disease hugely influence well-being by changing how people feel, how well they sleep, their energy levels, and even the way they think. Even if you don't suffer from one of these conditions, the gut is still influential in your mental health. A healthy gut is a literal barrier against inflammation. In addition, fostering the right kinds of bacteria in the gut suppresses inflammation while helping maintain the integrity of the gut wall, and when high inflammation is strongly linked to depression, as well as less prefrontal cortex control, this can't be overlooked. To reiterate: **The way you think and feel — and in turn experience and respond to the world around you — is highly influenced by the health of your gut. And that is a direct reflection of your food choices.**

The Happy Chemical: Serotonin

The hormone that stands front and center in conversations about mood and depression is serotonin. We know it plays a role in regulating mood, and many antidepressants are thought to work in part by increasing serotonin levels in the brain. Serotonin serves many functions in the body and may also participate in other brain and mental health disorders, including anxiety, obsessive-compulsive disorder (OCD), post-traumatic stress disorder (PTSD), phobias, and even epilepsy. It's involved in appetite and digestion, bone health, sex, sleep, and even psychedelic experiences. As mentioned, gut bacteria help us produce serotonin, and most of the body's supply of serotonin—around 90 percent of it—can be found in the lining of the stomach and intestines. Nine percent of our serotonin is found in blood platelets, where it plays a role in clotting. What that means is that only 1 percent of the serotonin in the human body is found in the brain! But don't let that statistic fool you: serotonin is extremely important for healthy cognitive functioning.

There are at least fourteen different receptors in the brain for serotonin, all of which serve different purposes. The serotonin-1A receptor has been the most studied, and it has been closely linked to psychiatric disease—specifically, anxiety and depression. For example, the antianxiety drug buspirone and the antidepressant vilazodone specifically stimulate this receptor.

Typically, chemical receptors become less sensitive with repeated stimulation and therefore require increasingly higher levels of stimulation to be effective. We know this to be true with the insulin receptor, for example. Chronically high levels of insulin reduce the functionality of the receptor, leading to type 2 diabetes. This phenomenon also occurs with the dopamine receptor. It's why people need increasing levels of whatever the stimulant might be to get the same dopamine. But when it comes to the serotonin-1A receptor, we're still trying to figure out exactly how things work.

Serotonin is manufactured from the amino acid tryptophan. Tryptophan is considered an essential amino acid—the body cannot create it on its own. This means all the tryptophan in our bodies has to come from food. And therein lies a clear connection between diet and mood. Although it's yet to be confirmed by large-scale studies, a high-tryptophan diet has been shown to improve mood as well as lower cortisol release in response to acute stress.[44]

TRYPTOPHAN-RICH FOODS	
Sesame seeds	Turkey
Sunflower seeds	Spinach
Flaxseeds	Chicken
Pistachio nuts	Tuna
Cashews	Crab
Mozzarella cheese	Oats
Lamb	Lentils
Beef	Eggs

But when inflammatory chemicals are circulating at high levels in the body, the pathway that turns tryptophan into serotonin is altered. That is, inflammation steers the body toward production of other chemicals. Stress and increased levels of cortisol interfere in the same way. In these instances, tryptophan is diverted toward making a chemical called kynurenine. The increased activation of this kynurenine pathway has recently been implicated as a key link between inflammation and depression.[45] This may explain the strong correlation between inflammatory conditions such as metabolic syndrome, diabetes, and obesity and the increased risk of depression as well as between stress and mental health conditions.

In the presence of inflammation and/or cortisol, the kynurenine pathway is activated. Many studies have shown that the activation of the kynurenine pathway is indeed altered in people suffering from depression.[46] Some researchers feel that the activation of this pathway lowers serotonin levels, contributing to depression. However, more recent research reveals that the neurotic by-product of the kynurenine pathway might well be a bigger piece of the puzzle, causing negative downstream effects on mood.[47] While depression is known to be linked to abnormalities in the prefrontal cortex, new research suggests that metabolites of the kynurenine pathway are significantly correlated with reduced thickness in this part of the brain in people with depression.[48] Recent data also suggest that kynurenine pathway activation is linked to cognitive impairment in women with depression.[49] We're still figuring out how to harness this information to promote better mental health, but research into the kynurenine pathway, inflammation, and their connection to depression is intriguing and ongoing.

The Gloom in Glycation

Testing for metabolites of the kynurenine pathway is one way scientists have been able to connect inflammation to depression. However, in lab tests, we've been linking inflammation with mood for a long time. One of the most well-known markers of inflammation is C-reactive protein (CRP). And wouldn't you know it: high CRP levels correlate not only with severity of depression but also with a decreased connection between the reward circuit and the prefrontal cortex.[50] Considering that CRP levels are also highly elevated in obesity,[51] we see that poor diet, inflammation, and disconnection syndrome are closely intertwined.

We also want to discuss hemoglobin A1c (often called A1c), a marker of average blood sugar levels in the body over the course of several months, which is especially important in diabetics. A1c specifically reveals how much sugar is bound to a protein called hemoglobin, which carries oxygen in red blood cells. The higher the blood sugar, the higher the A1c. The process of sugar binding to hemoglobin is technically called glycation, and it matters because glycation leads to increased inflammation. In fact, there is a direct correlation between the blood test for A1c and inflammation.

So when you are looking at your A1c results, you're seeing a heck of a lot more than simply your average blood sugar levels. You're getting an indication of the level of inflammation in your body. We hope you can see the problem.

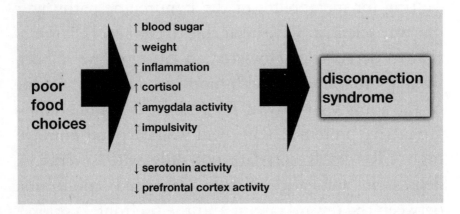

Let's take a closer look at the way inflammation affects your brain. One of the seminal longitudinal studies documenting the relationship between systemic inflammation and neurodegeneration has come out of the so-called ARIC study (Atherosclerosis Risk in Communities study), an ongoing study involving more than fifteen thousand individuals that began in 1987. The study was designed to examine risk factors for atherosclerosis by following people in four different communities over the years. It has allowed researchers to conduct various other types of investigations along the way, using the study's participants and their data. One such study was published in 2017 by a large group of researchers from multiple institutions, including

Johns Hopkins University, Baylor University, the University of Minnesota, and the Mayo Clinic.[52] The researchers measured markers of inflammation in a group of 1,633 individuals whose average age was fifty-three at the start of the study. They followed the participants for twenty-four years, assessing memory and brain volume as time progressed. Those who originally had the highest levels of inflammation markers had a significantly increased risk for brain shrinkage. In fact, their memory centers were 5 percent smaller in comparison to those who had lower markers of inflammation at the start. And if they had high levels of inflammatory markers, not only were their brains smaller, but their moment-to-moment brain function was also reduced. Indeed, after twenty-four years, the group with high inflammatory markers at the start of the study recalled the fewest words. These findings provide a powerful message for younger people who don't think about the way their habits — including things as simple as food choices — could be affecting their long-term brain health.

THE BRAIN WASH DIET

Given the information we have detailed in this chapter, it's clear that minimizing inflammation through diet is an important tool in reconnecting you to your prefrontal cortex. You will clear your table and bring back real foods for optimum thinking and brain power!

The diet protocol outlined in the ten-day plan starting on page 236 and the recipes starting on page 266 honor our ancestral roots, our genome, our microbiome, and our body's need for nutrient-dense whole foods from a diverse array of sources. The plan will help you reduce refined carbohydrates and added sugars, pushing your body to burn fat. Simultaneously, you'll increase your intake of healthful dietary fats. You'll consider "time-restricted eating" (more about this later) and eating at least one 100 percent plant-based meal a day, which will both lower your intake of pro-inflammatory foods and contribute to the sustainability of the planet. You'll be eating

- foods low in refined sugars and carbohydrates;
- non-GMO as much as possible;
- organic whenever feasible;
- fiber-rich, colorful produce (making up most of the plate);
- wild fish;
- grass-fed meat (if you choose to eat meat) and pastured eggs ("pasture-raised" eggs come from chickens that are allowed to wander outside, where they can eat what they would naturally eat in the wild, such as bugs, worms, and grass);

- modest amounts of gluten-free unrefined grains or seeds (e.g., wild rice, quinoa,* buckwheat,* and millet);

- healthful fats, including extra virgin olive oil, avocado oil, and nuts;

- probiotic-rich fermented foods;

- foods rich in prebiotic fiber, including dandelion greens, garlic, onions, leeks, and jicama (see the list on page 251);

- locally sourced foods; and

- more home-cooked meals.

You'll also be adding key supplements to your regimen, and we'll describe those in the ten-day protocol. We've created a delicious meal plan and plenty of recipes to help get you started.

Finally, we encourage you to plant a garden or even consider growing herbs or sprouts in a pot on a window-sill. Gardening reconnects us to the earth and to our food and, unsurprisingly, has been linked to a variety of positive health outcomes, including fewer depression and anxiety symptoms.[53] As you might expect, gardeners consume more vegetables than nongardeners. And when gardening is done in a communal setting, people are able to share ideas and generally connect with others. In fact, combining gardening with community is an

---

* Technically, quinoa and buckwheat are pseudocereals, not grains.

excellent way to bring together multiple positive steps to protect yourself from disconnection syndrome.

Food is one way you provide your body with the information it needs to reshape itself—from its neural connections down to its genetic expression. But there are other ways to effect change. What you do in your slumbering hours is another potent factor, and we will discuss this next.

CHAPTER 8

Sweet Dreams

The Overnight Brain Wash

Sleep is the golden chain that ties health and our bodies together.

—THOMAS DEKKER, ELIZABETHAN DRAMATIST

THOMAS DEKKER WAS RIGHT: SLEEP links our bodies to lasting health. Many people in fact have praised sleep through the centuries for its healing qualities. These writers appreciated the benefits of sleep a long time before we knew exactly what happens during the night and why slumber is so important.

How did you sleep last night? Did you get through the night without waking? Did you dream? Can you recall the last time you opened your eyes without an alarm in the morning and felt refreshed? If you can't call yourself a good sleeper, you're not alone. Fully one-third of American adults get less than the recommended seven hours of sleep a night.[1] That's a lot of people. Tens of millions of us. This is a national debt that needs our attention.

With so much competition for our conscious attention, it's little wonder we struggle to bank quality sleep on a regular basis. The electronic glow of digital screens illuminates our homes long after sunset. In place of natural light, we wake to the LED screens of alarm clocks or the blaze of our bright smartphones. Our circadian rhythms are subjected to all manner of assault, leading to fatigue and compromising our health. As doctors, we know sleep deprivation all too well. Medical trainees and practicing physicians pride themselves on their ability to function for more than twenty-four hours straight without sleep, albeit with the help of caffeine and power naps. We wear our sleep deficit like a badge of honor, but it contributes to myriad problems with memory, mood, and conditions as diverse as diabetes, excess weight, and dementia. It even contributes to early mortality itself. And as we'll explore in this chapter, not getting enough restorative sleep disrupts our ability to connect to the prefrontal cortex, making us more reactive and impulsive.

Scientists understand the value of sleep as they never have before. Laboratory and clinical studies have shown that virtually every system in the body, especially the brain,[2] is affected by the quality and amount of sleep we get. Sleep may influence how much we eat, what we eat, and how fast our metabolism runs. It influences how fat or thin we become, how well we can fight off infections, how creative and insightful we can be, how easily we cope with stress, how quickly we process information and learn new things, and how well we can organize and store memories. Most people don't appreciate how much of the body's inherent rhythm is grounded in sleep habits and controlled by the brain. Our body's natural day-night cycle—its circadian rhythm—has a hand in commanding everything about us, including our hormonal releases and gut microbiome. Even our gut bacteria know whether it's day or night and influence how we sleep.

Like our food choices, adequate sleep, which for the vast majority of us means at least seven hours each night, directly influences the expression of our DNA. In early 2013, scientists in England found that a week of sleep deprivation altered the function of 711 genes, including some involved in stress, inflammation, immunity, and metabolism.[3] Anything that negatively affects these important functions in the body also affects the brain. We depend on those genes to produce a constant supply of proteins to replace or repair damaged tissue, so it's critical that they function properly. Although we may not notice the side effects of poor sleep on a genetic level, we can certainly experience the observable effects: confusion, memory loss, brain fog, low immunity, obesity, cardiovascular disease, diabetes, and depression. All these conditions are uniquely tied to the brain.

Sleep problems play a large role in addictive behaviors, negative emotions, poor memory, and bad decision making. They diminish health and keep us from using our higher-order brains. On the other hand, good sleep is one of the most potent and undervalued tools for escaping disconnection syndrome. It's among the easiest, purest ways to reconnect to the prefrontal cortex. And it's free.

Sleep and the reason for its existence remained a mystery until the twenty-first century. Before we knew how important sleep was, it was easy to blow it off as an unnecessary luxury. Many people still claim they need only a few hours of sleep each night, though it's becoming increasingly clear that, by and large, these people are wrong. Despite the science, we cling to the idea that less sleep means we're able to get more things done by maximizing our productivity. We are encouraged to hustle, to get up early and grind until late in the night. This mentality has relegated sleep to a second-tier level of importance.

Once you gain an understanding of the way sleep affects you and your biology, our hope is that you make it a priority. (We won't go into the science of sleep from the perspective of its stages and "architecture" throughout the night; that's beyond the scope of this book. For a thorough look at sleep, though, we encourage you to read Dr. Matthew Walker's *Why We Sleep*.)[4]

WHY SLEEP IS KEY TO HEALTH

Scientists have been studying the way sleep affects the brain for some time now. In 1924, Cornell University psychologists John G. Jenkins and Karl M. Dallenbach noted that we preserve memories far better after we get a good night's sleep.[5] They state that "little is forgotten during sleep, and, on waking, the learner may take up the task refreshed and with renewed vigor." Since that time, our studies have become more advanced, but the results are no less compelling. Sleep is essential for storing memories. But we also now know that sleep plays multiple and diverse roles in brain functioning.

For example, it turns out that a sleep deficit will prevent you from processing information in general. Not only will you lack the ability to remember things, your ability to *interpret* information is also threatened. Sleep loss could be setting you up for *irreversible* memory issues, which in turn affect your mental processing and decision-making ability. An alarming 2013 study found that "Sleep fragmentation in older adults is associated with incident AD [Alzheimer's disease] and the rate of cognitive decline." Though we've known that disturbed sleep is a common aspect of neurodegenerative diseases like Alzheimer's, recent data show us that this sleep disruption may be present years before a person is diagnosed, suggesting that sleep problems may be an early marker of risk for dementia.[6] In other words, problems with sleep may be the first signal that something is going wrong in the brain.

Sleep deficits create issues throughout the body. A 2017 paper published by the American Heart Association showed that in patients with a history of heart disease, getting fewer than six hours of sleep was associated with a 29 percent increase in the risk of having a serious cardiac event (such as death or a heart attack).[7] A 2017 study of eighteen thousand adults showed that in prediabetics, logging fewer than six hours of sleep a night was associated with a 44 percent increase in the risk of developing full-blown diabetes, while getting fewer than five hours a night increased the risk by 68 percent.[8] The study concluded that "sufficient sleep duration is important for delaying or preventing the progression of prediabetes to diabetes." Remember that coronary artery disease, prediabetes, and diabetes are all inflammatory conditions. These diseases are strongly associated with worsened brain function and an increased risk of developing permanent cognitive decline.

In addition—and this is critically important—inadequate sleep will trigger the production of inflammatory chemicals,[9] which, through the kynurenine pathway we described in the previous chapter, are associated with depression and a relatively thinner prefrontal cortex.[10] In prediabetics and diabetics, it's a triple blow to the brain, because decreased sleep in combination with elevated blood sugar will further spark the glycation of proteins and the inflammatory storm that ultimately breeds chronic disease, depression, and disconnection from the prefrontal cortex—making happiness even more elusive.

Any conversation about sleep deprivation leads to a discussion about obesity. The number of studies documenting the relationship between sleep deprivation and weight gain and obesity could fill this book and then some. It's no longer debated that running a sleep deficit will pack on the pounds. How so? Several effects conspire to push your weight up, from complex hormonal changes in the body that increase appetite to an intense craving for junk food. According to one study, in sleep-deprived individuals, "neural changes were associated with a significant increase in appetitive desire for weight-gain promoting (high-calorie) food items following sleep loss, the magnitude of which was proportional to the subjective severity of sleep loss across participants."[11] In other words, foods that promote weight gain are consumed in direct relation to the amount of sleep deprivation one experiences. In 2011, the *American Journal of Clinical Nutrition* put a number on the increased caloric intake that results from sleep deprivation: three hundred extra calories a day.[12] Those calories add up.

How does sleep deprivation affect brain circuitry? As it turns out, sleep deprivation appears to cause overactivity of the amygdala and deactivation of the prefrontal cortex, increasing the chances for poor, impulsive food choices.

This research was taken a step further in 2019, when

researchers imaged the brains of people who had been sleep-deprived and compared them to those of people who had a normal amount of sleep.[13] In the sleep-deprived group, the amygdala was more actively communicating with the hypothalamus—the part of the brain that regulates hunger.

We have long recognized the strong association between sleep loss, nonrestorative sleep, and obesity, but now we understand why: *sleep deprivation robs us of our ability to make wise food choices.* Most of us can relate to this. Think of the last time you underslept. You likely craved foods high in sugar. It is exactly these unwise food choices that threaten the connection to the prefrontal cortex. The link between inadequate sleep and disconnection syndrome is clear.

If having better control over your dietary choices and your weight is not enough to inspire you to get a

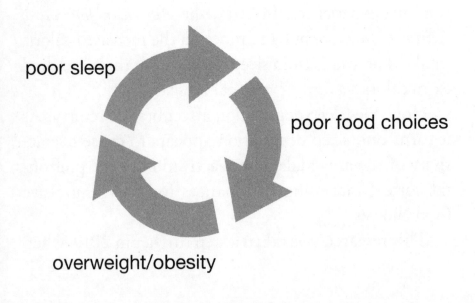

poor sleep

poor food choices

overweight/obesity

good night's sleep, consider what sleep deprivation does to the immune system. Have you ever caught a cold when you haven't had restful sleep? You'll recall that one of us (David) developed chicken pox, mumps, and dysentery during his medical residency, a time of incredible sleep deprivation (see page 28). There's a reason: sleep deprivation makes you susceptible to infection because it puts a damper on your immune system. The mechanism is twofold: important immune system cells that combat infections are diminished, and inflammatory molecules are increased. Not the condition you want to be in during cold and flu season. There's evidence that extremely serious sleep deprivation can be fatal. Rats deprived of sleep eventually die—their immune systems are compromised to the point where they succumb to an opportunistic infection.[14] And if sleep deprivation increases your chances of developing an infection, imagine what it's doing to your risk of suffering from other types of illnesses.

Sleep deprivation increases the risk of all the following through a complex combination of biological pathways.

- Excess weight and obesity
- Insulin resistance, metabolic syndrome, and diabetes
- Memory loss, confusion, and brain fog
- Dementia and Alzheimer's disease

- Lowered immune function
- Cardiovascular events, including heart attacks
- Cancer
- Low libido and sexual dysfunction
- Low mood and depression
- Susceptibility to infection
- Impulsivity
- Addiction
- Disconnection syndrome
- Shortened life expectancy

A TRUE BRAIN WASH

In 2012, Dr. Jeffrey J. Iliff and his team at Oregon Health & Science University published a paper describing a fascinating new discovery: the brain has a self-cleaning function.[15] This research sparked a new field of exploration into the drainage pathway that would come to be known as the glymphatic system — essentially a cleansing mechanism within the central nervous system that has been likened to a "shampoo for the brain" because it's responsible for removing molecular junk that builds up during our waking hours as part of the brain's normal metabolism. In 2013, another paper written by Dr. Iliff and colleagues, including Dr. Lulu Xie from the department of neurosurgery at the University of Rochester's Center for Translational Neuromedicine, proposed something equally interesting: the glymphatic system is much more active at night than it is during the day.[16] Sleep, it seems, provides a physical "brain washing." It not only helps us consolidate our memories and refresh our bodies but also appears to be key to the brain's housekeeping, allowing the overnight cleanup crew to do its job. Maybe this is why we spend a third of our lives asleep.

What happens when that waste is allowed to build up? Mounting evidence is showing us that this brain trash may be linked to an increased risk of developing dementia. In fact, even one night of sleep deprivation in humans is shown to be associated with an accumulation of one particular kind of brain trash called beta-amyloid, the brain protein that has been associated with Alzheimer's disease.[17] What's more, evidence now demonstrates a relationship between high levels of beta-amyloid accumulation and depression, especially in those with major depressive disorder who do not respond to treatment.[18] It also turns out that one of the brain areas targeted first by this amyloid buildup is the prefrontal cortex. In mice, this has been shown to disrupt the activity of the prefrontal cortex and block its ability to communicate with other parts of the brain.[19] We can agree that waste buildup anywhere—in our brains, in our bodies, in our homes, in our communities—does not create a healthy environment. We need adequate sleep to take the garbage out.

Unfortunately, as we grow older, this cleanup process may be harder to accomplish. One 2014 paper examined the ways in which the glymphatic system declines with age.[20] In mice, it was shown that there was a 40 percent decrease in the drainage rate in older versus younger mice. The implication for humans is that while we might not be able to reverse the effects of aging, we can focus on other ways to improve this process. Treating the sleep disturbances so common among old people is a good place to start.

> "It is difficult to imagine any other state—natural or medically manipulated—that affords a more powerful redressing of physical and mental health at every level of analysis."
> —Dr. Matthew Walker, *Why We Sleep*

Sleep's Mood Regulator

We've all experienced the painful day that follows a poor night of sleep. Feeling tired is rough. Perhaps you've noticed that you're more likely to snap at others and get annoyed or frazzled by daily challenges that you'd otherwise handle easily. This isn't coincidental.

Sleep is critical to our ability to handle emotional

stressors. By studying sleep's characteristic brain waves throughout its various stages during the night, scientists have shown that one stage in particular—REM sleep—is a key promoter of healthy emotional regulation. Even a quick REM-rich nap can help with this process. Researchers have made strides in figuring out why: sleep keeps the amygdala in check. In 2007, Dr. Seung-Schik Yoo and his team evaluated twenty-six healthy individuals between the ages of eighteen and thirty.[21] One group was able to sleep normally, while the other, less fortunate group was sleep-deprived for a full night. While undergoing fMRI brain scans a day later, both groups were shown images that were highly negative and designed to stimulate the amygdala. The people who were sleep-deprived experienced a 60 percent higher activation in their amygdalas compared to those who had a normal night's sleep. What's more, the researchers were able to demonstrate that the non-sleep-deprived group had a much stronger connection between the amygdala and the prefrontal cortex. The figure below shows that even one or two nights of missed sleep takes control away from the prefrontal cortex and gives it to the fear-based amygdala.

Bottom line: poor sleep may make us more emotionally reactive, detaching us from the ability to make rational, optimal decisions. And what are the downstream effects of this? Likely stress and an obesity-inducing diet, both of which in turn keep us from getting good sleep.

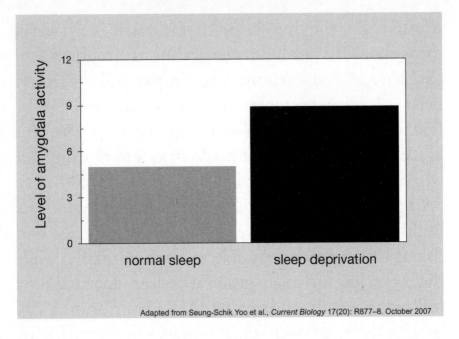

Adapted from Seung-Schik Yoo et al., *Current Biology* 17(20): R877–8. October 2007

In 2009, researchers proposed a central theory about the way sleep changes our brain activation to favor low emotional reactivity, explaining that "a night of sleep may 'reset' the correct affective brain reactivity to next-day emotional challenges." How does it do this? By allowing the prefrontal cortex to suppress the amygdala.[22] Indeed, as stated by Dr. Andrea N. Goldstein and Dr. Matthew Walker in a 2014 paper, "without sleep, the ability to adequately regulate and express emotions is compromised at both a brain and behavioral level."[23]

This means more than getting impulsive, unnecessarily annoyed, or angry. A 2017 study found that depriving men of sleep for two days led to worsened anxiety symptoms compared to men who slept well—and the sleep-deprived men showed an amygdala–prefrontal cortex disconnect. Not surprisingly, the authors concluded that "having adequate REM sleep may be important for mental health maintenance."[24]

Part of the reason for this finding may lie in the way sleep changes our interactions with others. A 2018 study conducted by Dr. Eti Ben Simon and Dr. Walker showed that sleep deprivation led to social withdrawal. They hypothesized that this could increase loneliness. Their disquieting paper "[proposes] a model in which sleep loss instigates a propagating, self-reinforcing cycle of social separation and withdrawal."[25]

The take-home message is simple. If we want to face the world with the best chance of success, and especially if we hope to break free from the emotional instability of disconnection syndrome, better sleep must be part of the plan.

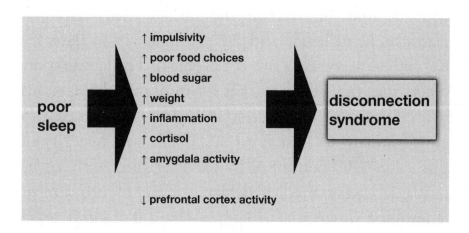

Sleep and Addiction

Given what we've discussed about sleep's effects on the brain, it's no surprise that sleep deprivation can influence the risk of addiction. And the scientific data speak to this. A 2010 paper looked at the association between sleep issues and relapse among drug and alcohol abusers, concluding that "sleep [disturbance] is a universal risk factor for relapse."[26] Given that impulsivity increases with poor sleep, this makes a lot of sense. For those who don't have a bona fide drug or alcohol addiction yet struggle with unhealthful foods, beverages, and even social media, sleep deprivation may make it all the more challenging to break the cycle.

SLEEP AIDS

America loves its easy fixes. Health-care providers and patients alike understand the burden that insomnia places on its sufferers, and the pharmaceuticals industry has rushed in to help solve the problem. The latest report shows that the global market for insomnia therapeutics was valued at $2.18 billion in 2016 and was predicted to grow annually at least until 2025. The vast majority of this value—99 percent of it—is drug sales, with 1 percent attributed to medical devices.[27] Every month, almost ten million Americans will pop a sleep aid of some sort.[28] People will do anything to get a better night's sleep. Given that so many of us are using these medications, it's reasonable to ask whether they work and if they're safe to take.

First and foremost, there is no reason to take any medication unless it works. That might sound self-evident, but think of the following: a scientific review in 2012 compared common sleep medications to placebos and concluded that "the [differences between the] drug effect and the placebo response were rather small and of questionable clinical importance."[29] It would seem we're not getting much bang for our buck. But wait — there's more.

Popular sleep medications can cause significant health consequences that last much longer than a single night. These pills can make it challenging to be productive the next day. Taking these medications also may increase your risk of cancer, depression, infections, and dementia. More important, these drugs appear to increase your risk of dying early. When more than thirty thousand adults were followed over the course of two and a half years, those taking the most hypnotics (prescription sleep medications) had a 530 percent increased risk of death compared to those who didn't take the drugs.[30] Sleep medications have been linked to around four hundred thousand US deaths per year.[31] Dr. Daniel Kripke of the University of California at San Diego was one of the first to extensively study the dark side of sleeping pills, finding that "the number of hypnotic-associated deaths may be almost comparable to the number of deaths attributed to cigarette smoking, cancer, or heart disease."[32]

With all this said, taking a sleeping pill may make it *seem* as though you've gotten more sleep or at least a better night's rest. But no type of sleep aid, whether an over-the-counter formula or prescription, induces natural sleep. Sedation is not the same as sleep. Granted, there may be a benefit to taking a short-term prescription sleep aid under the guidance of a doctor, and there may be a time and place for sleep-promoting supplements such as melatonin and valerian root, which is derived from an herb. But natural, pill-free strategies to improve your sleep hygiene will likely outperform everything else in the long term.

GOT SLEEP?

You may not even be aware that you have poor sleep quality. If you find that despite getting enough sleep you're still tired during the day—especially if you are male, overweight, have high blood pressure, or have been told you snore—talk to your doctor about your sleep. He or she might suggest you consider a sleep study, known technically as a polysomnogram. This is a painless, noninvasive procedure during which you spend a night in a sleep facility. As you sleep, a technologist records multiple biological functions to determine if you have any disorders such as sleep apnea or restless leg syndrome. When these conditions are treated, your sleep, your health, and the quality of your life will radically improve.

You'll want to find a certified sleep physician who is approved by the American Board of Sleep Medicine. Another great resource for sleep-related information in general is the National Sleep Foundation (www.sleep foundation.org).

THE BLUE-LIGHT BLUES

Why aren't we sleeping? In the nineteenth century, the invention of the electric light heralded a new age in sleep. Night no longer necessarily meant darkness. These days, the break between day and night has become blurry, even invisible, thanks to the inescapable spread of this artificial illumination. Far from the days when we relied on candlelight, we now discuss light pollution and its effects on natural cycles. And it's not just the amount of light: it's also the color. The blue-light-enriched LED screens we're constantly looking at are clearly having an impact on the quality and quantity of our sleep. Blue light is not blue per se — it refers to a certain wavelength of light on the spectrum of visible light that has effects on us through our eyes. This type of light stimulates us, boosting attention and reaction times. It's beneficial during the day, when we want to be awake and alert, but can sabotage us at night.

A major way in which blue light ruins our sleep has to do with melatonin. Melatonin is a hormone that plays a crucial role in helping our bodies prepare for a night of sleep. This hormone tells the body that it's time to shut down for the night and helps regulate circadian rhythms. Unfortunately, melatonin production can be significantly affected by light exposure at night. This may explain why looking at an e-reader—or any digital screen, for that matter—before bed diminishes the quality of sleep and lowers alertness the next day.[33] One study showed that even small amounts of light exposure at night could suppress melatonin production in the body and affect your circadian rhythm.[34] (Melatonin is available in supplement form, as noted above. But taking a melatonin pill is not the same as letting your body produce it naturally.)

Light exposure at night may mean more than poor sleep. New research indicates that exposure to light at night can increase the risk of certain cancers. In one trial, men who slept in illuminated bedrooms had an almost threefold increase in the risk of prostate cancer compared to those sleeping in the dark.[35] Nighttime exposure to the type of blue light that emanates from tablets, phones, and screens has also been associated with an increased rate of breast cancer in women.[36] In animal trials, blue-light exposure at night seems to induce depressive symptoms and lower expression of the crucial protein BDNF.[37]

With all this in mind, it's important to take a critical look at where we're focusing our attention before bed. Nearly half of American children use screens in the hour before they sleep.[38] A 2006 poll of American adolescents showed that 97 percent of those surveyed have at least one electronic item (TV, phone, music-playing device) in their bedrooms and that twelfth graders have around four of these devices.[39] Cell phones, tablets, TVs, and computer screens are all sources of blue light.

LIGHT THERAPY: IT'S ALL ABOUT TIMING

Although you'll want to limit your exposure to blue light before bed by minimizing screen time and keeping electronics out of the bedroom (or by wearing blue-light-blocking glasses if you must be in front of a screen), it helps to let natural sunlight (which does contain blue light) shine in in the morning. Early morning light will reset your body's clock naturally by traveling through your eyes to the suprachiasmatic nucleus, a tiny part of your brain that serves as the central pacemaker for your circadian rhythm.

On a positive note, several companies are now developing technologies to help mitigate some of the harm posed by nighttime light exposure. For example, many devices now support a "night mode," which reduces blue light. A 2018 study shows that wearing amber blue-light-blocking glasses in the evening versus clear lenses may improve the quality of sleep.[40] Some data even suggest that the negative effect of light before bed can be reduced with exposure to bright light in the morning.[41] As part of the Brain Wash ten-day program, we give you the tools you need to manage your night-time light exposure. We also provide tips to help you get better sleep. Elevated blood sugar can also be a sleep thief, but through the Brain Wash diet protocol you'll gain control of this important aspect of your health. Good sleep is essential for a happy, healthy brain, and it's high time we recognize this fact.

CHAPTER 9

Happy Body, Happy Brain

A Body in Motion Stays in Motion

If you are in a bad mood, go for a walk. If you are still in a bad mood, go for another walk.

—Hippocrates

It's no secret. We all know we should be exercising more. We know that exercise helps with weight control, strengthens our muscles and bones, reduces the risk of disease, increases self-confidence, and improves our outlook on life. These benefits are no longer headline news.

What is rarely talked about in the mainstream, however, is that **exercise rewires and restructures the brain for better functioning and higher-order thinking.** Few people think about the effect of exercise on the way we think, behave, make decisions, and relate to people. It's time to change that.

Science has sparked a revolution in our understanding

of why our bodies—and, specifically, our brains—need exercise to thrive. In this chapter, we'll explain how staying in motion can help you reclaim your cognitive circuitry for lasting health and happiness. Exercise, and movement in general, is a fundamental component of the Brain Wash program because, like sleep and food, it directly manipulates DNA expression while restoring your connection to your prefrontal cortex.

For millennia, exercise and movement were intrinsic, crucial components of daily life. Hunter-gatherers had no choice but to forage and hunt for nutrition, relying on their feet for transportation. The more we moved, the fitter—and bigger—our brains became, and the more we built tightly knit communities, shared resources, and depended upon one another in multifaceted social constructs.

In the past, evolutionary scientists liked to draw parallels between our foraging skills and our ability to engage in complex social interaction, since both these activities demanded complicated thinking patterns. But now scientists are proposing that physical activity itself may have shaped our brains into advanced thinking machines. Anthropologists have examined connections between brain size and endurance capacity in animals.[1] They looked at species ranging from guinea pigs and mice to wolves and sheep, noting that the animals with the highest innate endurance capacity also had the highest brain volumes relative to their body size. Then the researchers looked at mice and rats that were intentionally bred to be marathon runners. Levels of BDNF and other substances that promote tissue growth and health were increased in these specially bred animals, leading scientists to conclude that physical activity might have helped us evolve into clever, quick-witted beings with big, multilayered brains. **Our exceptionally complex and especially large prefrontal cortex — and therefore our ability to empathize, love, create conscious, thoughtful intention, feel compassion, and exist as high-performing beings — may stem largely from our physical prowess.**

Which raises the question: What happens to us when we become sedentary beings? Studies show that the prefrontal cortex is preferentially activated by exercise.[2] Forgo exercise, and we forgo the gifts of the prefrontal cortex and, as a result, grow ever more self-centered, emotionally unstable, isolated, anxious, and depressed. We become unfit physically and mentally. And we worsen disconnection syndrome.

Though we've moved from the African plains to industrialized cities, our bodies' needs are the same today. Our brains' healthy functioning requires regular physical activity regardless of how old we are. The simple act of moving your body will do more for your brain than any crossword puzzle, math equation, or mystery book. Research going back decades and ongoing has shown that exercise improves brain function, cognition, and plasticity—the ability of the brain to form new connections and reorganize itself. Exercise even acts as a "first aid kit" for damaged brain cells. We don't know of a single pill that can do all that for you. Moreover, exercise reduces inflammation,[3] reduces insulin resistance,[4] and at moderate, well-balanced levels helps keep cortisol in check[5] (unless you're trying to complete an Ironman triathlon, but that's another story). Collectively, these positive effects help the prefrontal cortex modulate the amygdala's response to incoming sensory data. In short, exercise helps reestablish important connections in the brain.

But we no longer need to search the woods for sustenance or migrate to greener pastures when food runs low, and as our bodies settle into computer chairs, recliners, and plush sofas, the metabolic stressors and physical demands that helped keep us healthy vanish. Modern technology has afforded us the privilege of a sedentary, relatively isolated existence: virtually anything we need these days is available without our having to exert much effort or even get out of bed. We get nowhere near the recommended amount of daily exercise. When you think about it, it's not all that strange that we feel an aversion to exercise because, as Harvard evolutionary biologist Daniel Lieberman states, "humans evolved to be adapted for regular, moderate amounts of endurance physical activity into late age," but "humans also were selected to avoid unnecessary exertion."[6] In essence, our bodies are designed to exercise regularly, but our energy conservation system is designed to save calories. Call it the exercise paradox. We are simultaneously wired to move and to avoid expending excess energy.

This has created a health crisis in today's world. Exercise reenergizes the brain in a way that nothing else can, sparking growth and potentially stemming the tide of neurodegenerative disease and mood disorders.

We could write hundreds of pages about the benefits of exercise. Instead, we'll drill down to some of the lesser-known effects of movement on the body.

THIS IS YOUR BRAIN ON EXERCISE

In the United States, around 8 percent of adolescents get the recommended sixty minutes of exercise daily, and only 5 percent of adults get the recommended thirty minutes.[7] Americans spend more than half the day in a sedentary state. We're far from our ancestral average: data from modern-day hunter-gatherer tribes, such as the Hadza indigenous group of Tanzania, show that a daily foraging trip equates to walking approximately 5.5 kilometers (3.4 miles) for women and approximately 8.3 kilometers (5.1 miles) for men.[8] What is our idleness doing to us?

A lot of media have covered the "sitting is the new smoking" angle. And for good reason: a 2015 meta-analysis and systematic review published in the *Annals of Internal Medicine* showed that sedentary behavior was linked to premature death from all causes.[9] In addition, movement itself is shown to *prevent* illness and death. A 2015 study that evaluated people over a period of several years, for example, revealed that getting up from a chair every hour for two minutes of light activity was associated with a 33 percent reduction in the risk of dying prematurely of any cause.[10] And in many large-scale analyses, physical activity has been shown to lower the risk of many types of cancer, including colon cancer, breast cancer, endometrial cancer, and meningioma (a type of brain tumor).[11] How so? Likely, at least in part, through exercise's wonderful controlling effect on inflammation. When you have less chronic inflammation, you lower the chance that cells will go rogue and turn into cancer.

Exercise and Executive Function

If the general health benefits of exercise aren't exciting enough for you, get this: exercise improves cognition. As we previously stated, executive function allows us to turn conscious thought into deliberate action — to bring our past experiences to bear on current decisions, experience the present with purpose and true depth of emotion, and frame today's actions in terms of potential future consequences. Strong executive function is a reflection of a healthy prefrontal cortex. And a healthy prefrontal cortex requires exercise.

A 2003 meta-analysis of studies on the relationship between exercise and cognition in the elderly showed that "fitness training was found to have robust but selective benefits for cognition, with the largest fitness-induced benefits occurring for executive-control processes."[12] Exercise affords us the opportunity to take control of our actions and ultimately make better choices, such as which foods to eat, when to shut off the TV at night, when to get outside into nature, where to focus our attention, and whether to continue to exercise.

In 2011, a randomized trial looked at the effects of exercise on the brain function of overweight children.[13] A total of 171 kids between the ages of seven and eleven were selected for the study. Children who exercised scored significantly better than those who did not on tests of executive function, planning, and math. They also had significantly increased blood flow to their prefrontal cortices. A similar study conducted in 2017 looked specifically at the way high-intensity training affected cognition in children.[14] High-intensity training involves short bursts of hard exercise, usually cardio. In this study, 310 children between the ages of seven and thirteen either did ten minutes of high-intensity training five days a week for six weeks or played board and computer games and took quizzes. The kids who engaged in exercise enjoyed significant improvements in cognition and, in particular, memory. Another 2017 study looked at adults with mild cognitive impairment, which is generally considered a precursor to full-blown dementia, and asked them to do either aerobic activity or stretching for six months.[15] Follow-up imaging showed that the aerobic exercise group had more coordinated activity across the prefrontal cortex. In other words, the prefrontal cortex lit up. In 2019, yet another study, led by a Duke University group, reached a short but informative conclusion: "Aerobic exercise promotes improved executive functioning in adults at risk for cognitive decline."[16] Doesn't this make you want to get up and move right now?

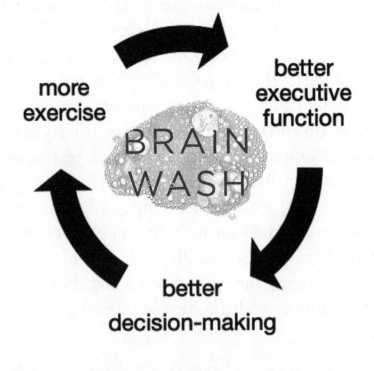

Biologically, then, exercise seems to increase blood flow to the prefrontal cortex, shuttling over more nutrients and helping it grow stronger. Meanwhile, connections to the prefrontal cortex become more robust. This is neuroplasticity at its finest, and it's sending a clear message: if you want a cognitive edge, exercise is essential.

Social Movement

In addition, if exercise helps us access and strengthen the prefrontal cortex, and if a strong connection to the prefrontal cortex is essential for empathy, it stands to reason that exercise should help us connect with others and enhance our empathic behavior. This hypothesis has yet to be confirmed in research, but it follows from the available information. And depending on the circumstances, exercise could be a wonderful way of reconnecting with nature and even getting some sunlight. Something as simple as catching up with a friend during an afternoon walk can be of benefit to health.

Exercising with a partner has been shown to improve adherence to a consistent exercise regimen. When people make plans to exercise together, their brains and bodies reap the benefits. In one study, older adults (men and women between the ages of sixty and ninety-five) were given information on ways to incorporate exercise into their lives. After four weeks, it was seen that "in participants whose partners took part in the

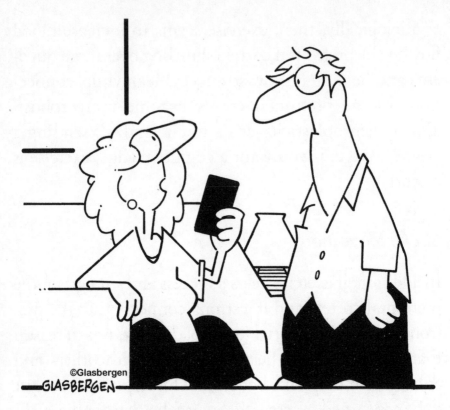

**"I guess I should start exercising again.
My treadmill sent me a friend request!"**

intervention, physical activity increased substantially over time, whereas it did not change in those individuals whose partners were not involved in the intervention, and it did not change in singles."[17] And when a large meta-analysis of nineteen studies and around 4,500 participants looked at whether walking with others helped improve exercise, it found that "interventions to promote walking in groups are efficacious at increasing physical activity."[18]

A Stronger Brain Through Exercise

Exercise not only changes the wiring and associated activity of the brain but also changes its physical infrastructure. Think about the brain's gray matter as the computer and its white matter as the cables that allow electrical signals to be transmitted. White matter is the way information gets quickly transferred from one part of the brain to another. When white matter is increased and more active, the brain's connections are fortified.

A 2014 trial showed that children who were physically in good shape had better development of white-matter communication pathways than those who were in poor shape.[19] Cardiorespiratory fitness was also correlated with increased white-matter activity in adults between the ages of fifty-five and eighty-two, implying that being in good shape might preserve brain function.[20] If exercise energizes and revitalizes the brain, might it also help prevent dementia and the associated decline of good decision-making skills? A 2018 study examined the frequency of white-matter hyperintensities (small spots seen on brain scans that may relate to Alzheimer's and vascular dementia) in people with various risk factors for cognitive decline.[21] It found that while white-matter hyperintensities increased with age, the increase vanished with higher levels of cardiovascular fitness.

Another 2018 study looked at patients with a high genetic predisposition to developing Alzheimer's disease and tracked their exercise habits as well as whether they developed the disease.[22] They found that those with high levels of physical activity did 3.4 times better on a cognitive examination and developed dementia more than fifteen years later than those who exercised less. The benefits conferred by fifteen extra years of clear thinking cannot be overstated.

Long-term studies can be the most revealing, especially when they span decades and follow large groups of people. One trial tracked 1,400 women who had completed a test of their cardiovascular fitness more than forty years earlier.[23] Rates of dementia were monitored at multiple points over the years. The results? In those who had high fitness levels compared to those with medium fitness levels, the risk of developing dementia was 88 percent lower. In those with low fitness levels compared to medium levels, the risk was 41 percent higher. This should give us serious pause.

EXERCISE AS AN ANTIDEPRESSANT

Given what we know about the consequences of untreated depression and the relative lack of effective pharmaceutical treatment options, it's vital that we consider other ways to manage the ailment. Exercise is finally getting the nod. In 2013, the rigorous reviewers at the Cochrane Library, which houses a collection of databases in medicine and other health-care special-ties, concluded that exercise is effective at helping reduce symptoms of depression.[24] A more current review of the available literature on depression and exercise in the elderly was published in 2016.[25] It exam-ined three meta-analyses and concluded that "exercise is safe and efficacious in reducing depressive symptoms in older people. Since exercise has many other known health benefits, it should be considered as a core inter-vention in the multidisciplinary treatment of older adults experiencing depression." And to be clear, not only is depression debilitating in its own right but, as we know, inflammation is also strongly associated with the condition's development.

It's good to know that exercise may be a safe and effective treatment for depression. But it's even more inspiring to think that it might *prevent* depression. A 2017 paper described a study that followed, for eleven years, approximately forty thousand adults who were free of any mental health diagnosis.[26] It found that reg-ular leisure-time exercise was associated with a reduced risk of depression. Based on the strength of this rela-tionship, the authors proposed that even one hour of physical activity a week could prevent 12 percent of future depression cases. Powerful therapy indeed.

These types of studies are correlative, not causal. This means we can't be sure whether depressed people tend to avoid exercise or if people who exercise only infrequently have a high likelihood of becoming depressed. But when a 2019 study conducted by researchers at Harvard University instead suggested that too little physical activity *causes* depression, it took the media by storm.[27] The study, involving hundreds of thousands of people, concluded that jogging for fifteen minutes a day (or walking or gardening for a little longer) can help protect against depression. The scientists used a cutting-edge research technique called Mendelian randomization, which provides evidence about causal relations between modifiable risk factors—in this case, amount of exercise—and a health issue such as depression. We won't get into the details of this kind of study other than to say that it's useful in finding cause-and-effect relationships in medicine that are otherwise hard to identify or prove. But the researchers' conclusion, that "enhancing physical activity may be an effective prevention strategy for depression," is revolutionary.

Although many factors play a role in the development of depression, no doubt at center stage is inflammation. Exercise's anti-inflammatory effects on the body have a profound impact on metabolism, hormonal cues such as cortisol levels, and brain function, including executive function and cognition powers—all of which affect your mood. **When you move, you put your prefrontal cortex in the driver's seat.** Ask regular exercisers if they feel connected to and in control of their bodies, and you will hear a resounding yes.

And choosing regular exercise becomes much easier once you begin to reconnect to that prefrontal cortex. Let your executive function lead the way.

FIND THE MOTIVATION

What if you hate exercise? How do you get yourself to do it? There's no easy answer, but you have to find your own motivators to get yourself off the couch. Some tips:

• Enlist the help of a friend and plan sessions together (e.g., go hiking or take a class). Again, this is like giving yourself a double dose of medicine. You're exercising. You're engaging in a real conversation with someone. And if you do it outdoors, that's a triple dose, because you've got nature in the mix.

• Join an online class, download an exercise video, or use an app that tracks your exercise habits.

• Lay out your workout clothes before bedtime and plan to exercise first thing in the morning.

• Schedule your workouts a week in advance and block them out on your calendar. Commit to your schedule. You will never *find* time for exercise if you don't *make* time for it.

• Consider taking a vitamin D supplement (more on this in the ten-day plan). Data show that it may help exercise performance, and that may further inspire you to stick with your regimen.[28]

We'll give you more ideas for prioritizing exercise during the ten-day plan. But start small and build up time and intensity in increments. All the research shows that you don't have to be a CrossFit champion or ultramarathoner to benefit from the power of exercise. As we said above, even getting up out of your chair for two minutes each hour can be helpful!

Although a small number of studies have found cognitive benefits among older people who lift weights, most studies, and all animal experiments, have involved running or other aerobic activities such as swimming, bicycling, hiking, and brisk walking at least five days a week for at least twenty minutes per session. We realize that exercise may not be on your list of top priorities, but we hope the evidence we've provided in this chapter will encourage you to rethink your daily to-dos. Exercise should include a mix of cardio, strength training, and stretching. Strength training and stretching will help you avoid injury and keep your routine, well, routine. If you don't have a regular workout regimen, it's time to set one up. If you already exercise, focus on increasing the duration and intensity of your workouts, or try something new.

Remember, a body in motion tends to stay in motion.

Once a body is in motion, other biological effects take place: less inflammation; lower stress and cortisol levels; better blood sugar control, insulin balance, and weight control; better sleep; better mood and memory; higher serotonin activity; greater activity in the prefrontal cortex; enhanced empathic behavior; less disconnection syndrome. It's a win-win all around.

CHAPTER 10

Quiet Time

Be Mind Full

Silence is a great healer. Let yourself block out the noise of the world from time to time and listen to your inner voice—it will tell you what you need.

—Anonymous

WHEN WAS THE LAST TIME you intentionally sat in silence for a few minutes? No distractions whatsoever. Nothing in your hands. Nothing within earshot or within sight to capture your attention. Was that moment earlier today? Yesterday? Can't even remember? You're certainly not alone. Let's try an experiment. For one minute, close your eyes and notice the thoughts that come up. They might seem incredibly random and disorganized. The chaos inside the modern mind is always there, ruining our ability to focus and remain present. Is it any wonder we're so frazzled and distracted?

As we've explained throughout this book, we're inundated with stimuli, often when we don't choose or want to be. In many respects, our time is no longer our own. The sacred, silent space in our minds reserved for reflection is shrinking. We need to reclaim this real estate for our health, happiness, and mental well-being. An inner sense of calm is the antidote to the frenetic modern world. Such stillness is readily available to you today, but you need to know how to receive it. It will help you take back your brain — wash it, rewire it, and protect yourself from disconnection syndrome.

Let's say you notice that your computer is running slowly. Thinking something is wrong with it, you turn to a computer expert. The first thing any technician would ask is how many applications you have open and how many programs are operating in the background. That's a good question to ask about your own brain. Because unlike the computer, you can't run multiple programs efficiently. The more you try to multitask, the more mistakes you make: one study showed that error rates were three times higher when participants were given two goals instead of one.[1] That computer technician, by the way, would tell you to update all your applications as well as your operating system, then do a cold hard reboot of your computer to refresh everything. We're asking you to do the same thing. That hard reboot will reset your mind for better, more efficient function.

This chapter shows you how quiet time allows you to start this upgrade today. When you make the choice to carve out quiet time for yourself—to *make* time, not occasionally find time—you will create a space for real personal growth. You get to decide whether you want your life to be dictated by others or under your control. Mindfulness and meditation practices directly oppose the idea of outside influence by putting you in charge of your mental processes. There's a reason so many have adopted these practices: they empower us all with the ability to change our brains.

The increasing popularity of research into mindfulness and meditation is a testament to this concept. Before the year 2000, the website PubMed listed fewer than ten studies a year on mindfulness. By 2019, that number had skyrocketed to more than six thousand. A search for studies on meditation shows a similar growth. And the general public has adopted these activities at an astonishing pace. In late 2018, the Centers for Disease Control and Prevention released a report on the rise of yoga and meditation among American adults, finding that from 2012 to 2017, participation in yoga increased 50 percent while engagement in the practice of meditation more than tripled, from 4.1 to 14.2 percent.[2] These practices share a common theme: pulling awareness back to the self. Here's why so many people are turning to these mindfulness practices: we desperately need them in our lives, and science clearly shows us the reasons.

The terms *mindfulness* and *meditation* are often used interchangeably, and definitions vary tremendously. For our purposes, mindfulness is a form of meditation. Mindfulness is about consciously directing your focus to a single thing and becoming aware of the present moment. Eating, walking, or deep breathing can therefore all become ways to practice mindfulness. So can prayer, certain styles of yoga, and progressive relaxation exercises. Meditation is more of an umbrella term for activities that focus on inward reflection and mental tranquility. There are many types of meditation. But mindfulness and meditation have the same goal: to calm the mind and create the space for reflection and grounding.

THE SCIENCE OF CALM

Mindfulness and other meditative practices such as deep breathing are powerful tools for wellness. We're learning that these types of focused activities are capable of changing the body's chemistry and physiology. For example, meditation has been shown to lower blood pressure.[3] A 2017 review of the effect of mindfulness on chronic pain concluded that "mindfulness meditation interventions showed significant improvements for chronic pain, depression, and quality of life,"[4] while another review revealed that mindfulness meditation, a specific type of meditation that emphasizes a focus on your present internal and external experiences, could improve the function of the immune system, largely through its effects on immune-boosting cells.[5]

Further research in this field has shown that mindfulness in general can reduce biological signs of system-wide inflammation, which as you know is associated with many diseases and, it's important to note, the brain's ability to think clearly and better employ the prefrontal cortex.[6] Meditation may even help prevent cognitive losses as we age: one review of the available literature stated, "Preliminary evidence suggests that meditation can offset age-related cognitive decline."[7] There's also evidence suggesting that mindfulness practices may present an effective treatment for insomnia.[8] Have we convinced you yet?

We often think of mindful activities such as yoga and meditation as methods to combat stress. This connection has been well substantiated. In 2014, for example, a group of marines received training in mindfulness-based techniques prior to being exposed to high-stress simulations of military activity.[9] The researchers found that the heart and breathing rates of marines who had received mindfulness training returned to their normal baseline levels faster than those of marines who had not received the training. The marines who had the training also showed signs of improved immune function. In fact mindfulness techniques are increasingly being used in the military. In 2019, army infantry soldiers at Schofield

Barracks, in Hawaii, began using mindfulness to improve their shooting skills. The practice can help a soldier avoid distractions amid chaos and focus on when to pull the trigger, avoiding unnecessary harm to civilians. In 2019, NATO held a two-day symposium in Berlin to discuss the evidence behind the use of mindfulness in the military. We predict it will become a staple in the training of soldiers.

You don't have to be a soldier to benefit from mindfulness and other forms of meditation, however. One of the most comprehensive and well-cited studies in this area, a meta-analysis published in the *Journal of the American Medical Association,* reviewed all relevant trials on the subject, finding that mindfulness significantly reduces anxiety, depression, and pain.[10] Another large-scale analysis looked at the effect of a practice called Transcendental Meditation on 1,295 people across sixteen studies.[11] It, too, found that such a practice led to significant reduction in anxiety, which became even more pronounced in those starting off with high levels of anxiety.

What is going on physiologically to produce these powerful effects?

How Mindfulness and Other Forms of Meditation Change the Brain

Mindfulness techniques give you a way to consciously regain control over your thoughts, allowing you to rewire your brain for mental balance and happiness, creating connections where they matter most and giving you the tools to deal with the stressors of modern life. They can put you back in the driver's seat in your own head. How do they change your brain?

A 2011 study conducted at Harvard University showed how effective mindfulness can be on influencing the brain's structure.[12] In this study, images of participants' brains were obtained using high-resolution MRI. Then half the participants completed an eight-week training program called mindfulness-based stress reduction. Compared to those who did not participate in the training, this group experienced significant increases in gray matter concentration across multiple parts of the brain after completing the course. Their brains were visibly and quantifiably different.

This study built upon a seminal 2005 paper in which researchers at Massachusetts General Hospital, a teaching hospital of Harvard Medical School, published one of the first imaging studies to show that meditation is associated with increased thickness of the brain's cortex.[13] Since then, numerous studies have documented that "thick-brained" people tend to be smarter and have stronger memories than those with "thin" brains. And meditators tend to not suffer from the age-related brain loss seen in nonmeditators. Meditation may help preserve brain areas involved in attention, sensory processing, and planning complicated tasks or goals.

Most impressive is the fact that it may not take much mindfulness to change the brain. A 2010 study showed that eleven hours of mindfulness practiced over a one-month period was sufficient to create measurable changes on brain scans.[14] And how might this brain rewiring be happening? One way is that meditation amps up the brain's BDNF.

What does it look like when these interventions are taken to an extreme? In 2011, researchers at Yale University enlisted meditators who had logged, on average, more than ten thousand hours of practice over the course of their lives.[15] They compared brain scans of the expert meditators with those of healthy nonmeditating volunteers. The results showed that meditators had significantly less activation of what's called the default mode network—the region of the brain that is thought to be responsible for mind wandering—than nonmeditators. In other words, meditation may help us to stay focused and present, escaping a mindless, distracted approach to the day.

Here's the key takeaway: because meditation reinforces areas of the brain that help us stay focused and present, **it helps reprogram our brains for well-being, empathy, and gratitude. It also acts as a shield against the ongoing efforts to hijack our brains, strengthening our ability to resist.**

As we've mentioned, our conscious actions and behaviors are largely regulated by the prefrontal cortex, which can analyze and act on information coming from the limbic system (containing the amygdala). In 2007, Dr. Yi-Yuan Tang and his colleagues at Stanford University's Center for Compassion and Altruism Research and Education examined whether meditation could affect this important bit of brain signaling.[16] They were able to show that five days of meditation training (for only twenty minutes a day) led to improved performance on a test of executive function. More recently, in 2015, Dr. Tang demonstrated that mindfulness meditation could improve the ability to control emotions and stress levels.[17] These improvements related to increased activity in the prefrontal cortex. The data dovetail perfectly with other trials showing that meditation enlarges the prefrontal cortices of meditators compared to the prefrontal cortices of those who only practice relaxation.[18]

In a time of rampant loneliness, it's also worth noting that meditation can increase our feelings of closeness with others. One study found that, in comparison to control subjects, a few minutes of loving-kindness meditation—a particular type of meditation designed to promote compassion and cultivate love—increased feelings of social connection.[19] The authors suggested that such a practical technique could help increase positive social emotions and decrease social isolation. It's unsurprising, then, that in meta-analyses meditation has also been shown to improve social emotions and behaviors.

Another research team wanted to test whether brain regions involved in executive function would also display increased connectivity after a mindfulness intervention. And indeed, they documented a significant increase in functional connectivity between the prefrontal cortex and several other regions of the brain after only three days of mindfulness practice.[20] Perhaps more fascinating is that a 2013 paper by the team's lead author showed that mindfulness was correlated with a smaller amygdala—the participants in the study group who were the most mindful had relatively smaller amygdalas compared to others in the group.[21] This was true even after the researchers controlled for age, total gray matter volume, neuroses, and depression. But while it's great to be calm and collected when we're meditating, what about the other parts of the day?

A 2012 study showed that many of the positive changes associated with meditative practices affect the way we process emotion. The authors found that eight weeks of training in two different forms of meditation "yielded distinct changes in amygdala activation in response to [emotionally charged images] while the subjects were in an ordinary, non-meditative state. This finding suggests that meditation training may affect emotional processing in everyday life, and not just during meditation."[22] In other words, maintaining a regular meditation practice can, essentially, permanently restructure the brain and enable it to better cope with the stressors of life.

One central goal of mindfulness and meditative practices is to reestablish brain connections so that we can use our high-level brain function to better navigate our lives and avoid the pitfalls that come from consistently viewing the world as a scary and dangerous place. This allows us to reconnect to others and to our own deep sense of meaning and wellness. It also has the potential to give us what's called ecological mindfulness. We now have scientific support for the idea that meditation inspires our efforts to solve complex environmental and sustainability challenges, including climate change. It can even motivate us to work for social justice and participate in activism. Put simply, when compared to nonmeditators, meditators care more not only for others but also for society at large and the planet. In the words of a 2018 paper published in the journal *Sustainability Science,* "It is concluded that mindfulness can contribute to understanding and facilitating sustainability, not only at the individual level, but sustainability at all scales."[23]

Given all these benefits of mindfulness practices, what are you waiting for?

AUSTIN'S MEDITATION PRACTICE

When I started my meditation practice, I was floored by the chaos inside my head. It was a real challenge to force myself to sit and observe this disorganized madness when I closed my eyes. It was almost as though my brain were trying to keep me distracted. But I understood that this inner disarray was a reflection of the way my mind was processing the world. It was the program that was constantly running in the background of my day-to-day life. With practice over time, I was less distracted by intrusive thoughts and better able to focus my attention.

Daily meditation, which I practice right after I wake up, has now become an essential tool for me. More than anything else, it helps me see how my mind is working each day—to see whether it's balanced and focused or distracted and moody. This insight lets me course-correct to improve my thinking, my decision making, and, in turn, my overall quality of life.

IT STARTS WITH THE RELAXATION RESPONSE

The body's innate relaxation response also plays a part in the effect that mindfulness has on our health. Consider deep breathing, for example. As we mentioned in chapter 6, when you perceive stress, the sympathetic nervous system springs into action, resulting in surges of the stress hormones cortisol and adrenaline. The parasympathetic nervous system, on the other hand, helps trigger a relaxation response. Deep breathing is one of the quickest means of inducing a parasympathetic response, flipping the switch from high alert to relative peace in seconds as your body calms down on many levels. According to the esteemed Dr. Herbert Benson, founder of the Benson-Henry Institute for Mind Body Medicine at Massachusetts General Hospital and among the scientists who first documented thicker cortical regions among meditators, the relaxation response is "a physical state of deep rest that changes the physical and emotional responses to stress." This state is characterized by:

- a slowed heartbeat,

- relaxed muscles,

- slower breathing, and

- a decrease in blood pressure.

Dr. Benson's institute pioneered the field of mind-body medicine and, in particular, the study of the relaxation response, a term he coined.[24] His work has even quantified the relaxation response's effects on gene expression before, during, and after long-term meditation routines. This research has been prolific and profound. For example, a 2013 paper written by Dr. Benson and his team showed that the relaxation response was linked to a lower expression of the genes involved in inflammation as well as stress-related pathways.[25] And it appears that the relationship between optimal gene expression and the relaxation response is linked to dosage: more relaxation means increased benefit. It's worth noting, too, that beneficial changes in gene expression were seen within minutes, after only one session. The Benson Institute scientists theorize that the biological events that take place during meditation essentially prevent the body from translating psychological worry into physical inflammation. This helps explain why mindfulness-based meditation practice has been shown in randomized trials to improve depressive symptoms in patients with chronic pain[26] and to have lasting antianxiety effects[27] after only eight weeks of group practice.

THE BENEFITS ASSOCIATED WITH MEDITATION

- Increased connection to the prefrontal cortex
- Better decision-making ability
- Increased sense of connectedness and empathy
- Improved relationships
- Higher levels of BDNF
- Better memory
- Reduced inflammation
- Reduced cortisol
- Reduced stress
- Improved creativity
- Improved cardiovascular health
- Better immune function
- Better control of blood sugar
- Improved sleep
- Greater concern for the health of the planet

TWELVE MINUTES A DAY

Dr. Andrew Newberg is the director of research at the Marcus Institute of Integrative Health–Myrna Brind Center and a physician at Thomas Jefferson University Hospital.[28] He has published more than one hundred articles and essays. His research has included studying meditation as well as people's spiritual experiences and attitudes. When we reached out to Dr. Newberg to ask about his research on meditation and memory, he was kind enough to forward several interesting publications written by members of his group. In one paper he reveals that putting individuals with memory problems on an eight-week meditation program resulted in a significant increase in blood flow to the prefrontal cortex as well as other areas of the brain.[29] Even the participants' memory function improved. In another study, fifteen individuals with memory loss (average age: sixty-two) were enrolled in an eight-week meditation program.[30] Upon completion of the program they underwent a neuropsychological test that showed "notable improvement trends in mood, anxiety, tension, and fatigue," with the relief of tension and fatigue being the most significant. All these trends correlated with changes in blood flow to the brain. And here's the kicker: the meditation technique required only twelve minutes a day.

If you're resistant to the idea of learning meditation, you can start with practicing moments of silence. A fascinating 2015 paper looked at the growth of new brain cells in the memory center—the hippocampus—under conditions of silence.[31] Compared to mice exposed to noises, mice that were placed in silent conditions for two hours a day had increased growth of brain cells in their hippocampi. In humans, one study showed that when researchers paused a song they had been playing, the resulting period of silence led to substantially lower heart rate and blood pressure in their subjects.[32] If you cannot recall the last time you sat in silence without distractions, it might be time to build more of those moments into your routine. Eventually you can work your way toward mastering meditation or another mindfulness practice.

As a final incentive, we need to emphasize that these practices work by helping us observe our thoughts and our behaviors. They provide insight by exposing our impulsive and emotionally reactive tendencies, allowing us to recognize how, when, and why these responses take hold and dictate our actions. The awareness that results from this understanding is one of the biggest goals of the Brain Wash program and is a fundamental outcome of engaging the prefrontal cortex.

As with a lot of the suggestions we make in this book, these meditation practices are free and do not require any special equipment. They don't need to be performed in a traditional manner—by chanting in the lotus position, say—and you don't have to concentrate on an object until your eyes dry out. Nearly every religious tradition practices a form of meditation, of which prayer is only one. There are many easy ways to practice mindfulness and other forms of meditation that will lead to impressive results without requiring you to spend the rest of your life in a cave. You can go to a class or download an app such as Headspace or Calm and be mindful at home. You can start with something as simple as listening to a guided meditation for a few minutes a day and working up to twelve minutes twice a day. A wide range of styles and methods of applying meditation to modern life are available, so there's no excuse. Below is at least one exercise you can try right now.

DEEP BREATHING

Deep breathing can be done anywhere, anytime. If you've never meditated before, a deep breathing practice twice daily will get you started.

Sit comfortably in a chair or on the floor. Close your eyes and make sure your body is relaxed, releasing all tension in your neck, arms, legs, and back. Inhale through your nose for as long as you can, feeling your diaphragm and abdomen rise as your stomach moves outward. Sip in a little more air when you think you've reached the top of your lungs. Slowly exhale to a count of twenty, pushing every breath of air from your lungs. Continue for at least five rounds of deep breaths.

Remember, meditation is not about achieving perfect enlightenment. The process (and all the challenges that come with it) fosters insight and perspective. We all have intrusive thoughts throughout the day, even during meditation. It's part of the human experience. Don't feel discouraged if meditation is challenging at first for you: that's the way it is for everyone!

CHAPTER 11

The Ten-Day Brain Wash

Putting It All Together

The secret of getting ahead is getting started.

—Attributed to Mark Twain

Welcome to the ten-day Brain Wash. This is a reset for your brain and body. Its purpose is to help you to reclaim your health and joy by giving you back control over your thinking, decision making, and behavior. You will transform your habits, your relationships, and the way you experience your life. It starts with just ten days of focused effort. You can do this.

Let's begin with a few core principles. First, you have to want to change for this to work. If you're content with an impulsive, disconnected lifestyle, and you don't mind all the damaging effects it imposes on your physical and mental health, this program isn't for you. Second, you shouldn't expect that this will immediately solve all your problems. **This is not a quick fix.** We're giving you a blueprint for long-term success and the permanent recalibration of your mental machinery.

The ten-day plan is designed to be as practical as possible without sacrificing benefits or testing your willpower to an unrealistic extreme. It is not a call for perfection but instead a kickoff to big changes in your life. We know that you may have many demands on your time and resources, but we ask that you do your best to make the most of these ideas and begin the ten-day plan when you know you can fully commit to it.

Each element of the plan works with the others to help your brain break free from disconnection syndrome while building your body's resilience and resistance to disease.

At the end of ten days, the fundamentals of the program should be continued indefinitely, but you can choose which additional components are most helpful for you to carry forward. This is the start, not the finish. By day 10 you will have established a new rhythm that you will continue to shape day after day.

THREE GROUND RULES

You're about to start a life-transforming journey. We want to make sure you're prepared for the path ahead. Here's how to set yourself up for success.

1. Be Honest: Success on the program requires you to be truthful. That includes taking a hard look at your health, your use of technology, and your diet. You'll also need to be frank about your cravings, your impulsive tendencies, your bad habits, your emotional control, your relationships, and the overall quality of your life. Though life is complicated, unpredictable, and constantly challenging, you are fully capable of making the necessary changes to build a body, brain, and life you love.

2. Commit: We won't downplay the fact that this plan may be a real challenge. Monumental transformations in wellness should be hard! You might struggle with some aspect of the program. We get it. No matter what kind of commitments you already have, you can build this into your life. Remember, these changes ultimately have the power to radically shift your long-term well-being for the better. This plan represents *freedom*. Freedom from body-weight chaos, chronic inflammation, pain, anxiety, low energy, and feeling lonely, helpless, and out of control. Freedom from disconnection syndrome. Each of the first eight days focuses on one particular area of your life.

- Day 1: Digital interactions
- Day 2: Empathy
- Day 3: Nature exposure

- Day 4: Diet
- Day 5: Sleep
- Day 6: Exercise
- Day 7: Meditation
- Day 8: Relationships

On days 9 and 10 you will evaluate your progress and make a plan for the path ahead. By then you will have incrementally added eight new habits into your daily routine and reached the point where you are committing to

- applying the test of T.I.M.E. to all digital activity (see chapter 4),
- taking three to five minutes a day to practice empathy,
- finding thirty minutes once a week for nature exposure,
- following the Brain Wash–approved diet (see chapter 7),
- following the Brain Wash guidelines for successful sleep (see chapter 8),
- exercising thirty minutes a day,
- meditating twelve minutes a day, and
- taking ten minutes a day for interpersonal connection.

If you cannot commit to the above, this plan is not for you. Come back to the program when you're ready. We also should note that you can modify this plan to match your needs, slowing it down when necessary. For example, if you need an extra day to enact the dietary component (day 4), that is okay. We are asking, however, that once you begin, you continue the steps outlined all the way to completion. In addition, you may substitute any of the days of the program (from 1 to 8) for another, but we recommend against it unless a major conflict arises.

3. Find what works: We've generalized the core components in a way that works for the majority of readers. With that said, it's key to identify your own needs before, during, and after the ten-day plan. You might, for example, have no problem limiting your social media use and getting out into nature, but you may struggle to cut refined carbohydrates, ultraprocessed foods, and soda from your diet. The important thing is to recognize where you need extra help. To this end, we recommend keeping a journal of the things you find easy and, conversely, hard. Track your progress and document as much as you can. You can use that information to create a customized long-term plan. We'll also provide additional assistance in troubleshooting specific challenges (and the parts of the plan we struggled with) on our website, BrainWashBook .com.

DAY 1: THE DIGITAL DETOX

First and foremost, you need to create barriers between your brain and the incessant influence of digital distraction. This requires striking a new balance. The idea is not to completely cut technology out of your life. Instead you will overhaul your use of digital devices. You will get what you need from technology while limiting its ability to hijack your time and your brain. This is where the test of T.I.M.E., which we outlined in chapter 4, comes into play. On day 1 of the program, do the following:

1. Review and turn off nonessential notifications (push notifications, badges, email notifications, and others) on your smartphone and computer. This frees your mind for more meaningful tasks.

2. Review and delete unnecessary applications from your phone.

3. Make the "do not disturb" feature on your phone and computer the default option.

4. Start using airplane mode during meals and important conversations as well as while you're sleeping.

5. Set up your devices to limit their interference with your sleep. Turn on the night-mode function to cut back your exposure to sleep-disrupting blue light in the evening, or, if you don't have this functionality, download a third-party night-mode app that helps cut out blue light at night.

6. Determine whether social media is essential for your business and personal life. If not, plan to abstain from using it or substantially limit your time on these platforms. If it is necessary for you to maintain a social media presence, determine the minimum amount of time you need to accomplish your goal and schedule it into your day.

7. Create and adhere to specific time periods during the day for responding to text messages, emails, and phone calls, if possible. Be strict with these boundaries (see our T.I.M.E. tool reminder below).

8. Start cutting back on your TV viewing. This is a great opportunity to catch up on books, conversations, and, yes, even technology such as audiobooks and podcasts that encourage mindfulness and cognitive growth.

9. Cut out nonessential online shopping.

REMEMBER TO GIVE EVERYTHING THE TEST OF T.I.M.E.

We highly recommend employing the T.I.M.E. framework for social media use, TV viewing, internet browsing, online shopping, smartphone scrolling, emailing, and even responding to text messages. Manage your digital exposure by remem-

bering the four characteristics of healthful digital activity
(see chapter 4 for details):
Time restricted
Intentional
Mindful
Enriching

DAY 2: PRACTICING EMPATHY THROUGH GRATITUDE

Reflecting on the positive aspects of your life and the
people you care about is an exercise in mindfulness and
empathy, and studies show that more gratitude means
more empathy.[1] On day 2, write down five things you
are thankful for. These can be as specific as a delicious
meal or conversation with a friend or as general as your
good health. Put a journal, a notepad, or just a sheet of
paper as well as a pen or pencil by your bedside. You'll
spend a few minutes in the morning or evening writing
down five points of gratitude from this day forward. In
addition, make a daily goal of thanking someone in
person for something specific that individual has done.
This type of prosocial behavior helps you *and* the person you're thanking. As an optional step, take time
each day to pause and consider why someone who
holds a dissimilar perspective from yours thinks and
feels that way. This will further bolster your empathy
for others.

DAY 3: NATURE THERAPY

We understand that most people don't live within walking distance of an expansive forest. That's fine. Instead, the idea is to do what is possible given your individual circumstances. Researchers are still determining exactly how long people need to be in nature to reap its benefits, but in the meantime, we're asking you to spend at least thirty minutes today somewhere in nature. You do not have to go to extremes. Start by locating parks and green spaces near you; nature is readily available to all of us if we just get outside. Even in an urban environment, the benefits of nature can easily be enjoyed. If you have no other options, you can simply walk outside your office or home and observe the landscape. Check out these resources (as well as others at BrainWashBook.com):

• The Outbound Collective (TheOutbound.com) has an incredible collection of outdoor recommendations.

• NatureFind.com has a good repository of nature destinations near you and lets you search by the activity you'd like to do (e.g., biking, fishing, and so on).

• RootsRated.com, like NatureFind, offers suggestions for outdoor experiences.

Once you've found a way to get out into nature, you may be a little unsure how to proceed. There's no one right way to forest bathe, as long as you're mindfully engaging with nature. Don't worry too much about accomplishing a specific goal. Instead, just try to take in the sounds, sights, and smells of the plants around you, using all your senses. Consider walking slowly and taking time to appreciate nature's diversity and complexity, whether you're at the beach, in a park, or walking around your neighborhood. Find a specific part of a park that appeals to you and spend extra time savoring the section you enjoy most.

Nature therapy lends itself to being combined with other Brain Wash recommendations because there's so much you can do outdoors. Think about meditating in a park or bringing a friend with you so you can bond over a picnic. You might even bring a book to read, a sketch pad, or a journal. Some parks host classes in mindfulness practices such as tai chi and yoga. The point is to be present in the moment and open to taking in the many benefits of being in nature. This means silencing your phone or turning it to airplane mode (or, better yet, leaving it in the car) and giving your full attention to the natural beauty around you.

As an additional step, consider buying houseplants to enhance your indoor environment. For most people, this means placing a plant next to a window in your home or office. Find a spot where you'll be able to enjoy the plant throughout your day. Try plants that are easy to take care of, such as succulents. Bring the outdoors in as much as possible.

DAY 4: FIGURING OUT FOOD

Dietary change has to start in the places where you have the most control: your kitchen and pantry. Now is the time to take a good look at what you've been eating—and get rid of everything that is hurting your health. While it's easy to make exceptions (such as saving those cookies and cans of soda for guests or keeping the cereal "just in case"), this is the moment to embrace the word *no*. Processed foods such as refined carbohydrates directly threaten your ability to use your prefrontal cortex. Remember, food is information for your body, all the way down to its neural networks, cellular connections, and genetic expression. You need high-quality nutrition to keep you thinking clearly.

General Guidelines

Use the rules we set forth in chapter 7 (page 176) to begin crafting your Brain Wash meals. As a reminder, try to eat more single-ingredient, plant-based foods. When considering packaged food in general, avoid consuming products that have more than five ingredients. That certainly doesn't mean you cannot cook with more than five ingredients. But avoid using or consuming artificial or processed ingredients that you wouldn't normally include in home cooking.

If you choose to eat meat, treat it as a condiment

instead of the main event. And make at least one meal a day, such as lunch, 100 percent plant-based (no meat or other animal-derived products). Also aim to build more probiotic- and prebiotic-rich foods into your day.

What to Eat

For a full list of the foods to toss or keep, visit our website at BrainWashBook.com. Below is an abbreviated list.

Toss

- All forms of processed, refined carbs, sugar, and starch, such as chips, crackers, cookies, pastries, muffins, pizza dough, cakes, doughnuts, sugary snacks, candy, energy bars, ice cream, frozen yogurt, sherbet, jams, jellies, preserves, juices, sports drinks, soft drinks, soda, sugar (white and brown), and corn syrup.

- All artificial sweeteners and products made with artificial sweeteners. Evict even the sugar substitutes that are marketed as "natural." These include the following: acesulfame potassium (e.g., Sunett, Sweet One), aspartame (e.g., NutraSweet, Equal), saccharin (e.g., Sweet'N Low, Sugar Twin), sucralose (e.g., Splenda), and neotame (e.g., Newtame).

- Be cautious about sugar alcohols that are marketed as healthful alternatives to natural and artificial sugars. These include ingredients such as sorbitol, mannitol, xylitol, maltitol, erythritol, and isomalt. We don't know yet what these could be doing to your microbiome and, in turn, your brain. It is known that sugar alcohols are often associated with gastrointestinal issues such as diarrhea and bloating.

• Processed meats, such as bacon, sausage, ham, salami, smoked meat, canned meat, dried meat, hot dogs, corned beef, and cold cuts. Most processed meats contain additives that can ultimately cause inflammation.

• Margarine, vegetable shortening, and most commercial brands of vegetable cooking oils (e.g., soybean, corn, cottonseed, canola, peanut, grapeseed, sunflower, and rice bran)—even if they are organic. These oils typically come from plants, but they are often refined and chemically altered. Their worst attribute is their high content of inflammatory omega-6 fats.

• Nonfermented soy products (e.g., tofu and soy milk) and processed foods made with soy (look for "soy protein isolate" in the list of ingredients and avoid soy cheese, soy burgers, soy hot dogs, soy nuggets, soy ice cream, and soy yogurt). Note that soy products that are fermented—including natto, miso, and tempeh—are acceptable; they provide a source of protein for vegetarians and are suitable for 100 percent plant-based meals. The main problem with unfermented soy is phytic acid, which reduces absorption of nutrients such as calcium, iron, magnesium, and manganese. It also contains lectins, which may increase inflammation and the risk of developing food allergies. Fermentation reduces these issues. Ideally, choose products displaying the non-GMO label.

• Foods containing ingredients that sound like chemicals or are otherwise foreign to you, such as maltodextrin, sodium nitrite, and sodium benzoate.

• Packaged foods labeled "fat-free" or "low-fat." Often, foods that emphasize their low-fat content as a way of appealing to consumers contain a significant amount of added sugar.

Keep

In place of these toxic products, purchase healthful real foods (most of which don't come with nutrition labels). Remember, go organic, non-GMO, and local with your whole-food choices wherever possible; flash-frozen is fine, too. Make a shopping list that includes colorful vegetables as well as healthful fats such as avocados, extra virgin olive oil, nuts, and seeds—and if you choose to eat animal products, consider buying sardines, mackerel, anchovies, salmon, or herring (a.k.a. SMASH fish) to improve your omega-3 intake. (For a downloadable sample shopping list, see BrainWash Book.com.) Look over the recipes starting on page 266 and mark a few you'd like to try, then add the ingredients to your shopping list. Below is a quick summary.

- **Healthful fats:** Extra virgin olive oil, sesame oil, coconut oil, avocado oil, organic tallow and butter from grass-fed cows, ghee, coconuts, olives, nuts and nut butters, and seeds (flaxseeds, sunflower seeds, pumpkin seeds, sesame seeds, and chia seeds).

- **Low-sugar fruit:** Avocado, bell pepper, cucumber, tomato, zucchini, summer squash, eggplant, lemon, lime.

- **Protein:** Plant sources of protein, including cooked legumes (e.g., black beans, kidney beans, pinto beans, fava beans, navy beans, lentils, peas, and chickpeas) and fermented, non-GMO soy products, such as tempeh and miso. Note that cooking is far more effective than soaking to reduce phytic acid and lectins in legumes. Animal sources of protein include pastured whole eggs, wild fish (sardines, mackerel, anchovies, salmon, and herring), shellfish and mollusks (shrimp, crab, lobster, mussels, clams, and oysters), grass-fed meat, free-range poultry, and wild game. Remember, meat should be treated as a condiment, not as the mainstay of your meal.

- **Vegetables:** Leafy greens, including lettuce, collards, spinach, kale, and chard; also broccoli, cabbage, onion, mushrooms, cauliflower, brussels sprouts, artichoke, alfalfa sprouts, green beans, celery, bok choy, radishes, watercress, turnips, asparagus, garlic, leeks, fennel, shallots, scallions, ginger, jicama, parsley, water chestnuts, celery root, kohlrabi, and daikon.

• **Probiotic-rich fermented foods:** Kimchi, kefir, cultured condiments, and live-culture yogurt.

• **Prebiotic-rich foods:** Dandelion greens, garlic, onion, asparagus, leek, jicama, and sunchoke.

The following can be consumed in moderation ("moderation" means eating small amounts of these ingredients once a day):

• **Starchy vegetables:** Beets, corn, potatoes, sweet potatoes, and yams.

• **Gluten-free grains:** Amaranth, buckwheat, rice (brown, white, and wild), millet, sorghum, teff, oats, and quinoa. Note that even though these are gluten-free, they are high in carbohydrates.

• **Cheese, cottage cheese, non-live-culture yogurt.**

• **Cow's milk (whole) and cream:** Use sparingly in recipes or in coffee and tea.

• **Sweeteners:** Natural granulated stevia and dark chocolate (at least 80 percent cacao).

- **Whole sweet fruit:** Berries are best; be extra cautious of sugary fruits such as apricots, mangoes, melons, papaya, bananas, pineapple, and dried fruit.

- **Wine:** One glass a day if you so choose, preferably red, low alcohol (12.5 percent or less), and organic.

Be mindful when you're eating. Remove distractions and focus on the food — how it tastes and feels as you consume it. Lastly, modify your eating schedule. Research on time-restricted eating and metabolism indicates that limiting your meals to a twelve-hour window can improve insulin sensitivity, blood pressure, and immune function. And, most relevant to our message, it lowers inflammation. Time-restricted eating supports the body's healthy circadian rhythm, too (for more on this topic, see our website and check out Dr. Satchin Panda's terrific book *The Circadian Code*). Further, research shows that it's best to avoid consuming anything but water in the three-hour period before bed.

Prepare yourself for the inevitable challenges posed by food. Though you may be able to control your food choices at home, things get complicated when you find yourself far from your kitchen. It's vital that you're ready for these situations. One way to plan ahead is to always carry a high-quality snack (a bag of nuts is a great option). Equally important, you'll likely experience instances when people around you are eating and drinking things excluded in the Brain Wash plan. Lunchrooms and workplace cafeterias, for example, are notoriously filled with junk food and other unhealthful enticements. You're going to have to decide if you'll allow yourself to bend to temptation or if you'll stay committed to the plan. Remember, that desire to cheat is the very reason you're doing this in the first place. Giving in is hand-delivering your reward center exactly what it needs to stay in charge.

Making lasting dietary change is one of the most challenging and meaningful aspects of the ten-day Brain Wash. You're certainly in good company if you struggle to maintain healthful eating habits. Don't forget to plan meals with friends, too. Catch up over a healthful breakfast or host a potluck dinner. However, remember to do your homework and keep the food options within the Brain Wash protocol. Below is a sample menu for a day followed by a list of four supplements to consider.

A BRAIN WASH SAMPLE MENU

Upon waking: Tall glass of warm water with optional squeeze of lemon and/or slice of fresh ginger

Breakfast: **Avocado Toast** (page 281) with optional **Powerhouse Coffee** (page 342) or green tea

Lunch: **Vegetable Lasagna** (page 314) with **Hibiscus Tea** (page 340)

Snack: **Matcha Smoothie** (page 338) or raw veggies such as celery and bell peppers cut up and dipped in **Cauliflower Hummus** (page 290)

Dinner: **Whole Roasted Salmon with Sunchokes and Leeks** (page 313) and a glass of red wine (optional)

Dessert: **Almond-Coconut Biscotti** (page 334) with a cup of chamomile tea

Remember: Avoid consuming anything but water within three hours of bedtime

Four Supplements to Consider

We haven't mentioned supplements with any frequency because we'd prefer that you get everything you need from "nature"—from the food you eat. But there are a few gems we'd like to highlight that can significantly support your body and brain during the Brain Wash program and beyond. You can pick them up at any high-quality market or online and start taking them today. For details about these supplements, visit our website at BrainWashBook.com.

• *Vitamin D:* Your body naturally manufactures this vitamin when sunlight hits your skin, but many people are deficient in it because of a lack of adequate sun exposure (they either live in northern latitudes, spend too much time indoors, or use sunscreen to block the UV rays needed to make this important vitamin). Overweight people tend to need more vitamin D than others to achieve healthy levels in the bloodstream—between 40 and 60 ng/ml (nanograms per milliliter). A starting point is to take a supplement containing 2,000 international units (IUs) of vitamin D_3 daily, but you should work with a medical professional to find the dose that is right for you.

• *DHA (docosahexaenoic acid, an omega-3 fatty acid):* Perhaps no other brain-boosting molecule has received as much attention as docosahexaenoic acid. DHA is an important building block for the membranes surrounding brain cells, particularly the synapses, which lie at the heart of efficient brain function. It helps reduce inflammation in the brain and throughout the body and appears to increase BDNF. Go with a dose of 1,000 milligrams (mg) daily. It's okay to buy DHA that comes in combination with EPA (eicosapentaenoic acid), which also serves to reduce inflammation. But check the DHA amount per capsule to be sure you're getting enough. Opt for a fish oil supplement or choose DHA derived from marine algae.

• *Turmeric:* Curcumin, the main active ingredient in the spice turmeric, is the subject of intense scientific inquiry, especially as it relates to the brain. It has been used in traditional Chinese and Indian (ayurvedic) medicine for thousands of years. Although it is well known for its antioxidant, anti-inflammatory, antifungal, and antibacterial properties, it is its ability to increase

BDNF that has attracted the interest of neuroscientists around the world. Go with a dose of 500 milligrams (mg) once daily.

• *MCT (medium-chain triglyceride) oil:* MCT oil is typically derived from coconuts. It is a form of saturated fatty acid that acts as superfuel for the brain—with the added benefit of reducing inflammation. Go with a dose of 1 tablespoon daily (preferably organic) or 1–2 tablespoons of pure coconut oil. And don't hesitate to cook with coconut oil or add MCT oil to coffee and tea.

DAY 5: SUCCESSFUL SHUT-EYE

Who would have thought that those hours of semiun-consciousness at night could be so valuable? The research on the health benefits of sleep is absolutely stunning (revisit chapter 8). You're going to use sleep to help reset your brain and put your prefrontal cortex back on top. There are three ways to prepare for successful sleep that you'll focus on.

• **Create a sleep sanctuary:** Make your room as quiet, peaceful, and sleep-friendly as possible. This means removing distractions (e.g., TVs, computers, phones, tablets, and so on). Hunt down and clear out any eye- and brain-stimulating electronics.

- **Set up for slumber:** Plan to cut out all caffeine after 2:00 p.m. Establish a bedtime routine that tells your body it's time for sleep. Even if you're not in your bedroom, limit all exposure to bright light within an hour of bedtime and use blue-light-blocking glasses if you must look at a screen in the evening. Maintain dim lighting around your home before bed, especially in your bedroom, and set the bedroom temperature between sixty-five and seventy degrees.

- **Wind down:** Just before bedtime, consider taking a warm bath or shower, listening to calming music, or reading a book. You can also write in your gratitude journal and meditate before lying down.

Consistent, high-quality sleep can be tough to come by. It might also take time to settle into a new sleep routine. Don't expect to get a perfect night's rest right off the bat, and remember that even a slightly higher quality of sleep is doing your health and your brain a great service.

DAY 6: EMBRACING EXERCISE

Getting consistent exercise may seem daunting. The idea is not to force yourself into something disagreeable but to see exercise as a form of medicine that preserves your brain and body while improving your mood and decision making. Use day 6 to focus on building this habit into your daily routine: make a move today by engaging in some form of exercise for at least twenty minutes. As you progress through the rest of the program, set a goal of upping that to thirty minutes a day. Below are the four keys to making exercise enjoyable.

• **Be realistic about your starting point:** If you haven't exercised in several years, you shouldn't get up and run for ten miles. The goal is sustainable movement!

• **Remove barriers:** Plan how and when you will exercise. Don't *find* time; *make* time. To that end, have your exercise clothes and shoes ready the night before.

• **Have fun:** Forcing yourself through the motions will be a lot less effective in the long run than finding activities that excite and energize you. Switch up your routine if it isn't working for you. Try a new activity if it keeps you motivated and moving.

• **Exercise with others:** Engaging in physical activity with others helps keep you moving. Try drafting a friend into your exercise routine for one day of the week. Consider joining a running or walking group. Ask a coworker if he or she would be interested in going for a walk at lunchtime. Active.com has a great assortment of local groups and activities (5Ks, hikes, and other suggestions) as well as a variety of helpful articles for those starting an exercise plan. Meetup.com provides a list of nearby group meetings, including walks and hikes. There's no excuse! Do what speaks to you and your body.

Once you reach your goal—a minimum of thirty minutes at least five days a week—you'll see that exercise doesn't have to be a dreaded task: instead, it can be a welcome part of your life. Even on days when you don't go through a regular exercise routine, think about building more movement into your day through little changes such as taking the stairs or going for a walk after lunch. If your job is relatively sedentary, get up and walk around for at least two minutes every hour: don't be caught sitting for hours on end. Eventually, you can ramp up your exercise by adding more intensity and time so that you achieve all the brain-nourishing benefits of BDNF and improved prefrontal cortex function. But don't forget that just moving—in any way—is wonderful for your mind and body.

DAY 7: MEDICATE WITH MEDITATION

As we explained in chapter 9, meditation is one of the best ways to debug your mind. We're not recommending a specific type of meditation because the main goal is just to make it part of your day—like exercise. You can learn about various styles of meditation online, get an instructional book, or download one of the recommended apps that we referred to on page 232. If you want to start with a basic technique that doesn't require technology, just sit and focus on your breathing for twelve minutes. Use day 7 to try one form of meditation and continue the practice daily thereafter.

Expect this part of the plan to challenge you significantly. Before you start, remember that it's completely normal for your mind to be distracted when you try to meditate. That's the whole idea! Catching your mind when it wanders is the goal, so don't feel like you're messing up when you lose focus. You'll need to find a time of day when you will have twelve uninterrupted minutes to spend meditating and a place where you won't be distracted. First thing in the morning or right before bedtime are excellent opportunities. You might consider investing in a meditation cushion, although a chair, couch, or even carpeted floor all work fine. You'll want to be sure to turn your phone on airplane mode or turn it off for the duration of your daily meditation, because digital intrusions will seriously interfere with the potential benefits of this activity.

DAY 8: STRONG BONDS

Your interactions with other people are key in helping you escape disconnection syndrome. You'll benefit from this activity by spending at least ten minutes of unbroken time connecting with another person each day. The catch: the connection has to take place in person or on the phone (or on a video chat), and it has to entail conversation dedicated to learning something new about the other person. On day 8, think about ways to make this effortless and ensure that the conversation takes up the full ten minutes. For example, you could have a sit-down dinner with your family and take turns sharing the best part of your day or what you learned. Consider calling an old friend you haven't spoken to in a while.

DAY 9: TAKING STOCK

How's it going? You might feel like you're just getting started, but now is the time to evaluate how the previous eight days went and where you want to go from here. Review any notes you've taken so far. What parts of the program were the most challenging? What has been relatively effortless? Have you gotten out into nature yet? Are you struggling to keep up with the digital detox recommendations? You probably have work to do in some areas, and that's okay.

Go over the following table and circle one option that describes how challenging each day has been for you. This will become a road map to tell you where you need to focus your efforts moving forward.

Day 1: Digital	Day 2: Empathy	Day 3: Nature	Day 4: Diet
Easy Medium Hard	Easy Medium Hard	Easy Medium Hard	Easy Medium Hard
Day 5: Sleep	Day 6: Exercise	Day 7: Meditation	Day 8: Relationships
Easy Medium Hard	Easy Medium Hard	Easy Medium Hard	Easy Medium Hard

Take some time to think about where your mental defenses were weak. Did you feel like you wanted to skip your workout at the end of a stressful day? Did you have trouble resisting free bagels at the morning meeting? Ask yourself what might have contributed to these situations. Think about how best to prepare for these moments (for example, signing up for an exercise class after work and eating breakfast before the morning meeting). This advance planning will help protect your brain and body.

Consider whether you're being manipulated when you invest your time, energy, and money in something that doesn't benefit you. Before you eat an unhealthful meal, binge on social media, or make the next impulsive purchase, for example, ask yourself whether you are acting in your own best interests or someone else's. Are others profiting from your poor choices? Use this insight as motivation to change.

Here's one more suggestion to try on this ninth day: write a letter to yourself to describe the reasons why you want to transform your life, and read it aloud each morning and evening. Find what most drives you and remind yourself repeatedly why you've made this investment in your future. Maybe you want to keep up with your kids, alleviate a serious health condition, lose weight, have a more intimate relationship with your partner, feel more energized and rested, or be more efficient and productive at work. When you write out your intentions and articulate them, you're more likely to maintain the habits that will ultimately help you realize your goals.

DAY 10: MOVE FORWARD

Bravo! You are on your way to a better life. You've begun to make significant changes that are affecting you right now on many levels, including your mood, metabolism, and brain function. Most important, you've started down the path of taking back your thoughts and actions—allowing you to break free from disconnection syndrome.

See if you notice any positive changes—for example, better sleep, fewer digestive issues, fewer cravings for sugar and junk food, more energy, relief from a chronic condition, or greater well-being in general. Take note of these observations, however small, and use them as fuel to keep you going.

The last step of this plan is to create a framework so you can continue to benefit from the lessons in this book for years to come. These ten days are meant for focusing on each technique one at a time, but you have to commit to them for life if you want to rewire your brain for lasting health and joy. It may feel impossible, but remember that incorporating even one of these recommendations into your daily routine is a major leap forward.

As you prepare to adopt the recommendations, consider the following three steps:

1. Review the chart from day 9 and focus specifically on the activities you found most difficult (the days you circled HARD). Go back and reread those sections of the book to see if there are ways to make these activities easier. In addition, visit our website (BrainWashBook .com) for further information on ways to overcome some of the most common hurdles.

2. Review the parts of the program that were most meaningful to you. Highlight the things that kept you energized, excited, and motivated and prioritize them as you create a sustainable plan for the future. If you find yourself growing tired of or less interested in any specific component, try switching things up (e.g., attempting a different workout, cooking different meals, exploring a new park, experimenting with a new type of meditation).

3. The ten-day Brain Wash asks you to make many changes. They may not all be relevant or viable for you. If you decide not to follow all our recommendations, we strongly encourage you to prioritize as many as possible of the core Brain Wash components.

- Apply the test of T.I.M.E. to all digital activities.
- Establish a daily practice of empathy.
- Spend thirty minutes a week in nature.
- Abide by the Brain Wash diet.
- Exercise for thirty minutes five days a week.
- Prioritize getting at least seven hours of sleep a night.
- Meditate for at least twelve minutes a day.
- Dedicate at least ten minutes a day to improving interpersonal relationships.

We hope you continue to practice the core fundamentals of this program every day, but we also hope you find ways to tailor the main ideas to your own life.

CHAPTER 12

The Brain Wash Recipes

Finding Connection in the Kitchen

WHAT YOU CHOOSE TO EAT and drink is one of the most important decisions you make each day. Food is a gateway for remodeling your brain and body. It is a ticket to a life of vibrant health and well-being. We've crafted original, deeply satisfying recipes that follow the Brain Wash protocol, including basics; breakfast dishes; appetizers, soups, salads, and small plates; sides, entrées, desserts, and drinks. These delicious anti-inflammatory menu options will fuel your body with the information it needs to optimize its overall function — supporting everything from the microbes in your gut to the neurons in your brain. Lots of these recipes are designed to be shared, so don't hesitate to double or triple them for a group get-together.

While you won't find any traditional breads, pastas, and pastries on the menu, there are plenty of delectable alternatives that won't feed your cravings for sugar and other addictive carbs. Remember, this is about cooking with fresh, whole ingredients that are as close to nature as possible. All the recipes in this book were tested using organic produce, pasture-raised or grass-fed poultry and meats, and eggs from pasture-raised chickens. Extra virgin olive oil, coconut oil, avocado oil, unsweetened nut milks, and fresh herbs and spices are also frequently used. If you don't have access to a farmers market, you can find all the ingredients at large supermarkets, chain stores, and specialty food stores as well as online.

Have fun with these recipes. Modify them as you see fit, but stay within the Brain Wash protocol. And if you're looking for more recipes, you'll find them online at BrainWashBook.com.

BASICS

Vegetable Stock

Makes about 6 cups
Time required: About 1 hour

There is nothing better than a nice, clean homemade broth or stock, even though you can buy fine-quality preparations at the store. For this vegetable stock, you can add and/or subtract any vegetables you want, but remember that strongly flavored vegetables, such as cabbage and broccoli, will add bold flavor to the finished product. We always add a piece of ginger for its healing properties.

3 medium organic onions, peeled and chopped

3 large organic leeks, including some green parts, trimmed, well washed, and chopped

2 organic carrots, peeled, trimmed, and chopped

2 cloves organic garlic, peeled and chopped

1 organic fennel bulb, trimmed and chopped

2 cups chopped fresh organic mushrooms

3–6 sprigs organic parsley

2 organic bay leaves

1-inch piece organic ginger, peeled

1 teaspoon organic black peppercorns

Fine sea salt to taste

Combine the onions, leeks, carrots, garlic, fennel, and mushrooms in a large deep saucepan. Add 7 cups water and stir to blend.

Add the parsley, bay leaves, ginger, and peppercorns along with the salt. Place over high heat and bring to a boil. Cover and lower the heat to a gentle simmer. Simmer for 30 minutes, or until the liquid is nicely flavored by the vegetables.

Remove from the heat and strain through a fine-mesh strainer into a clean container. Use immediately or let cool and store, covered, in the refrigerator for up to three days or in the freezer for up to three months.

VARIATIONS: To make mushroom stock, add 7 ounces of dried mushrooms to the above recipe along with the onions and other vegetables and simmer for about 45 minutes, or until the stock has a distinct mushroom flavor. Strain and store as directed.

To make poultry or meat stock, roast the backs and wings of pasture-raised chicken or turkey at about 350°F for about 30 minutes, or until nicely browned. Alternatively, roast the bones and a bit of stew meat from grass-fed animals at the same temperature for about 40 minutes, or until nicely browned. Add the browned chicken or meat to the above recipe along with the herbs and proceed as directed.

Leize's Basic Vinaigrette

Makes about 2 cups
Time required: About 15 minutes

Leize, wife and mother to us, has been making this vinaigrette since she learned the recipe from a wonderful French woman with whom she lived while in France many years ago. She now often just guesses at the amounts and makes the dressing directly in a wooden salad bowl. It is great to keep on hand for topping salads or even for drizzling on grilled fish, shellfish, pork, or poultry. It can also be made using avocado, coconut, or other nut oils.

1 small organic garlic clove, peeled and minced

2 tablespoons organic red or white wine vinegar

About ¼ teaspoon fine sea salt, plus more to taste

1½ teaspoons organic Dijon mustard

½ cup organic extra virgin olive oil

Freshly ground organic black pepper to taste

About 1 tablespoon chopped fresh organic herbs, such as basil, tarragon, parsley, or chives (optional)

Combine the garlic, vinegar, and salt in a small bowl. Set aside to mellow for about 10 minutes.

Using a whisk, beat in the mustard, then slowly pour in the oil, a bit at a time, whisking to emulsify. You may not need all the oil, depending upon how acidic you like your salad dressing.

Taste and season with additional salt, if necessary, and freshly ground black pepper. If using herbs, whisk them in just before serving.

Store in the refrigerator, bring to room temperature, and shake to blend before using.

VARIATIONS: Add 1 small peeled and minced shallot along with the mustard.

To make balsamic vinaigrette, replace the organic red or white wine vinegar with organic balsamic vinegar.

Aioli

Makes about 2 cups
Time required: About 12 minutes

Aioli sounds fancy, but it really is nothing more than a highly seasoned garlic mayonnaise. It is terrific as an accent for grilled or steamed vegetables, chilled poached fish or chicken, or poached or hard-boiled eggs. Because it is a kind of mayonnaise, it can also morph into a few other sauces that can broaden your repertoire.

2-3 threads saffron

1 tablespoon organic champagne vinegar or freshly squeezed organic lemon juice

3 large egg yolks from pasture-raised chickens, at room temperature

1 teaspoon smashed organic garlic

½ teaspoon fine sea salt

¼ teaspoon organic dry mustard powder

1½-2 cups organic extra virgin olive oil or avocado oil

Place the saffron in the vinegar and let it infuse for at least 30 minutes.

When ready to prepare the mayonnaise, fill the glass jar of a blender with boiling water and set it aside for a couple of minutes. The idea is to heat the jar to help the egg yolks thicken. Then pour out the water and quickly wipe the jar dry.

Add the egg yolks and blend on medium speed until very thick. Add the garlic along with the salt and mustard and quickly incorporate. Add the vinegar and process to blend. (You can either remove the saffron threads or leave them in. If left in, they will add a distinct yellow color to the finished product.)

With the motor running, begin adding the oil in an excruciatingly slow drip. The slower the drip, the more even the emulsion. When about half the oil has been added, you should have a sauce with the consistency of old-fashioned heavy cream, and you can begin adding the oil just a bit more quickly, because curdling will no longer be an issue. If the mixture seems too thick—you want a soft, creamy mix—add just a smidgen more vinegar. Continue adding oil until all of it has been absorbed into the eggs. Then, if necessary, add just enough hot water to smooth the mix, usually no more than a scant tablespoon.

Scrape the aioli into a clean container with a lid. Cover and refrigerate for up to five days.

VARIATIONS: Stir in 2 tablespoons chopped fresh herbs, minced green or red hot chili peppers, grated ginger, grated horseradish, or minced bell peppers to the finished aioli. Ground spices can also vary the flavor—cumin, cayenne pepper, and cracked black pepper are favorite additions. Turmeric and curry powder can give it a South Asian kick.

To make avocado aioli, add ½ cup mashed organic avocado along with the mustard and replace the champagne vinegar or lemon juice with freshly squeezed organic lime juice.

Brain Wash Dry Rub for Meats, Poultry, and Fish

Makes about 2 cups
Time required: About 15 minutes

This simple dry rub is a terrific way to introduce our favorite good-for-you spices into everyday cooking. It is quite potent but adds just the right amount of zest to grass-fed meats, pasture-raised poultry, or fatty wild fish such as salmon, particularly when grilled or roasted.

8 organic cardamom pods

3 whole organic star anise

3 2-inch organic cinnamon sticks

2-inch piece dried organic ginger root (see Note)

½ cup organic coriander seeds

¼ cup organic cumin seeds

¼ cup organic black or white peppercorns

1 tablespoon whole organic allspice

1 teaspoon whole organic cloves

1 teaspoon dried organic crushed red pepper flakes (optional)

Combine the cardamom, star anise, cinnamon sticks, ginger root, coriander and cumin seeds, peppercorns, allspice, and cloves in a medium frying pan over medium-low heat. Cook, stirring frequently and/or shaking the pan, for about 3 minutes, or until the spices are very fragrant and starting to color. It is important to keep the spices moving in the pan so they don't burn.

Remove from the heat and set aside to cool to room temperature.

When cool, place in a spice grinder, food processor, or blender and process to a smooth powder. If using, add the crushed red pepper.

Transfer to a glass container, cover, and store in a cool dark spot for up to six weeks.

NOTE: Dried ginger root is available at specialty food stores, health food stores, Asian markets, and online.

Ricotta Cheese

Makes about 1½ cups
Time required: About 2¼ hours

Homemade ricotta cheese is useful in so many ways. It can be eaten as a dessert, breakfast treat, or added to many dishes for extra creaminess and stability. It is also useful as a spread or as a component in salads. If you wish to use it solely as a dessert, you can add a teaspoon or so of stevia when you heat the milk.

- 2 cups organic whole milk from grass-fed animals
- 1 cup organic heavy cream from grass-fed animals
- ½ teaspoon fine sea salt (optional)
- 1 teaspoon granulated organic stevia, or more to taste (optional)
- 1½ tablespoons strained freshly squeezed organic lemon juice

Line the interior of a fine-mesh sieve with two layers of damp cheesecloth. Use pieces that are big enough to hang slightly over the edges of the sieve so that the mesh is completely covered. Set the lined sieve on top of a nonreactive container, such as a glass or stainless steel bowl, large enough to allow a few inches of space between the bottom of the sieve and the bottom of the bowl. Set aside.

Combine the milk and cream and, if using, the salt or stevia in a heavy-bottom saucepan over medium heat. Bring to a gentle boil and boil for 1 minute. Remove from the heat and stir in the lemon juice.

Set aside to rest for about 4 minutes, or just until the mixture separates into visible curds. Pour into the lined strainer, cover with plastic wrap, and set aside to allow the whey to drain for about 2 hours, or until the curds reach the desired consistency. The longer you allow the mixture to drain, the denser the finished cheese. Do not discard the whey; it may be used as a beverage or in any recipe requiring it.

Remove the plastic wrap, scrape the ricotta from the cheesecloth, and place it in a nonreactive container. Store, covered, in the refrigerator for up to five days.

Stone Age Bread

Makes 1 loaf
Time required: About 1½ hours

Variations of this bread exist all over the world. It is easy to make, exceedingly nutritious, a great alternative to white bread, and very filling. We always have it on hand and often share it with friends and neighbors as a delicious way to introduce them to the Brain Wash way of eating.

The one tool you'll need, which is useful for all sorts of recipes, is a kitchen scale. These are inexpensive and available online and in stores that sell kitchen supplies. You do not need to chop the seeds and nuts; use them whole, just as they are.

3½ ounces raw unsalted organic pumpkin seeds

3½ ounces raw unsalted organic sunflower seeds

3½ ounces raw unsalted organic flaxseeds

3½ ounces organic sesame seeds

3½ ounces raw unsalted organic almond slivers

3½ ounces raw unsalted organic walnut pieces

5 large organic eggs from pasture-raised chickens, at room temperature, lightly beaten

½ cup organic extra virgin olive oil

2 teaspoons fine sea salt

Preheat the oven to 325°F.

Butter a 9 × 5 × 3-inch loaf pan and line the bottom with parchment paper cut to fit. Butter the top of the parchment paper.

Combine all the seeds and nuts in a large mixing bowl. Add the eggs, olive oil, and salt and stir to combine completely.

Scrape the mixture into the prepared loaf pan. Transfer to the preheated oven and bake for about 1 hour, or until firm.

Remove the pan from the oven and let rest for 15 minutes. Turn the pan upside down and tap the bread out onto a cooling rack. Allow to cool slightly before cutting. Store in an airtight container in the refrigerator.

BREAKFAST

All-in-One Breakfast

Serves 2

Time required: About 7 minutes

This is easy and quick—and such a healthful break-fast. The greens, the avocado, the ginger, and the tur-meric give you all you need to get your day started on the right note. You can put the components together in the evening and pop them in the blender 1-2-3 in the morning.

- 4 sprigs organic flat-leaf parsley
- 1 large organic avocado, peeled and pitted
- 1 large leaf organic kale, trimmed of its tough stalk and chopped
- 1 cup organic baby spinach leaves
- 2 tablespoons organic mint leaves
- ½ teaspoon grated organic ginger
- ¼ teaspoon organic ground turmeric
- 2 cups organic coconut water

Combine the parsley, avocado, kale, spinach, mint, ginger, and turmeric in a blender. Add the coconut water and 4 ice cubes and process to a smooth puree.

Pour into two chilled glasses and drink up!

Almost Muesli

Serves 2
Time required: About 5 minutes

This mix has a bit more heft than the usual muesli and gives a warming welcome to a chilly morning. It is about as healthful a breakfast as we can imagine to start your day.

½ cup chopped raw unsalted organic almonds

½ cup organic hemp seeds

½ cup unsweetened flaked organic coconut

¼ cup organic oat flakes (see Note)

2 tablespoons raw unsalted organic chia seeds

1 tablespoon raw unsalted organic flaxseeds

¼ teaspoon organic ground cinnamon

⅛ teaspoon organic ground ginger

1½ cups unsweetened organic coconut milk

1 teaspoon MCT oil (see page 256)

½ cup organic blueberries

Combine the almonds, hemp seeds, coconut, oats, chia seeds, flaxseeds, cinnamon, and ginger in a small saucepan. Stir in the coconut milk and oil and place over medium heat.

Bring to a simmer and cook, stirring, for a couple of minutes, until the mixture has thickened.

Remove from the heat and spoon an equal portion into each of two small cereal bowls. Top with blueberries and serve immediately.

NOTE: Organic oat flakes, which are naturally free of gluten, are available at health food stores or online. Look for brands that have not been packaged in a facility that also processes wheat.

Avocado Toast

Serves 1

Time required: About 25 minutes

Although avocado toast seems to have been born in Australia, it is now served almost everywhere in the world. There are so many versions — some with just avocado, salt, and pepper, and some with many different components, including meat, fresh herbs, cheese, oils, and tomatoes. Just about anything you can imagine can be placed on top of the avocado, including a poached egg — our favorite. It's simple but delicious and a great way to start the day.

1 large egg from a pasture-raised chicken, at room temperature

1 teaspoon organic distilled white vinegar

1 small ripe organic avocado

1 teaspoon chopped organic cilantro

Juice of ½ organic lime

Fine sea salt to taste

1 slice toasted Stone Age Bread (page 276)

Organic crushed red pepper flakes to taste

Organic cilantro, organic mint leaf, or lime wedge for garnish (optional)

Pour about 3 inches of cold water into a small deep saucepan. Place over high heat and bring to a gentle simmer—you should see bubbles forming around the edge of the pan. Add the vinegar.

Break the egg into a small fine-mesh sieve placed over a small bowl, allowing the albumen to drip into the bowl. Transfer the egg to a small custard-style cup. This helps keep strands of egg white from forming in the water, resulting in a perfect round egg.

Stir the simmering water with the handle of a wooden spoon to make a slight vortex. Gently slide the egg into the center of the vortex. Simmer for about 2½ minutes, or until the egg white is firm and the yolk has just barely set.

Using a slotted spoon or spatula, carefully transfer the egg to a clean warm custard-style cup.

Split the avocado in half lengthwise and, using a

teaspoon, scoop out the flesh, discarding the pit. Place the flesh in a small shallow bowl and add the cilantro and lime juice. Season with sea salt and, using a kitchen fork, lightly mash.

Spoon the avocado onto the toast, smoothing the top slightly. Place the toast on a small plate.

Gently tip the egg from the warm cup into a slotted spoon. If the egg has strands of egg white dripping off the edges, carefully snip them off using kitchen shears.

Slide the egg on top of the avocado toast. Sprinkle a bit of crushed red pepper flakes over the top and garnish with a sprig of cilantro, a fresh mint leaf, or a wedge of lime if desired.

Breakfast Crepes

Makes about thirty 10-inch crepes
Time required: About 15 minutes

Although often served as a dessert—which you certainly can do with these almond-flavored delights—crepes make a wonderful breakfast dish, too. This is the Brain Wash take on the traditional French breakfast of bread and dark chocolate. It is a simple recipe, but you could also fill the crepes with scrambled eggs, berries, or grilled vegetables. You will need two nonstick 10-inch crepe pans (see Note), or you can cut the recipe in half and work with only one pan.

6 large organic eggs from pasture-raised chickens, at room temperature, lightly beaten

1½ cups organic almond flour

1 teaspoon fine sea salt

2–2½ cups organic unsweetened almond milk, at room temperature

3 tablespoons melted organic unsalted butter from grass-fed cows, plus more for coating the pans and serving

1 teaspoon pure organic vanilla extract

1 cup finely grated organic dark chocolate, at least 80% cacao

Break the eggs into a medium mixing bowl. Whisk in the flour and salt. Begin adding the milk in a slow, steady steam, whisking constantly. When you've added about half the milk, the batter should loosen, at which point you can add all the remaining milk along with 3 tablespoons of melted butter and the vanilla. The batter should lightly coat the back of a wooden spoon and have the consistency of half-and-half.

Preheat two nonstick crepe pans over medium heat. Lightly coat each one with melted butter. Using a small ladle, pour just enough crepe batter into one pan to coat the entire bottom. Take the pan off the heat and lift and swirl it until the batter has spread to evenly coat the bottom.

At this point, begin making another crepe in the other hot pan. Cook for about 45–60 seconds, or until the bottom is golden brown.

As each crepe is cooked, drizzle it with melted butter and dust with grated chocolate. Using a silicone spatula, gently fold the crepe in half, then fold the half into quarters.

Flip the folded crepe out onto a plate and serve as you repeat the above steps with the remaining batter.

NOTE: If you want to make the crepes in advance, place a parchment-lined cookie sheet in a 200°F oven. As each crepe finishes cooking, transfer it to the cookie sheet to keep warm. Do not stack; keep in a single layer.

When you make your first crepe, the batter might stick to the pan and tear when you attempt to turn it. This indicates that the pan has not been properly seasoned or that there is a bit of residue on it from past crepe making. Often, the first crepe (or even the second one) will stick because the pan is not at the correct temperature, but all subsequent crepes should pop right out. If the crepe looks as though it is pulling inward quickly, this indicates that the pan is too hot. If it doesn't set up almost immediately, the pan is too cold. All this sounds daunting, but it really does become easy once you get started.

Greens with Eggs

Serves 4

Time required: About 35 minutes

You can use any greens you like in this recipe. For variety and a stronger flavor, you might use dandelion and/or mustard greens or mix them in with the chard and kale. Since this takes a bit more work than the usual weekday breakfast, it is a suitable dish to serve on the weekend for brunch or lunch.

¼ cup organic extra virgin olive oil, divided

2 large organic leeks, white part only, trimmed, well washed, and thinly sliced crosswise

2 organic shallots, peeled and thinly sliced crosswise

1 large bunch organic Swiss chard, trimmed and shredded

1 bunch organic lacinato kale, trimmed of tough stalks and shredded

1 teaspoon minced organic garlic

1 tablespoon freshly squeezed organic lemon juice

4 large eggs from pasture-raised chickens, at room temperature

Fine sea salt and freshly ground organic black pepper to taste

1 teaspoon chopped fresh organic tarragon

½ teaspoon organic crushed red pepper flakes

½ teaspoon organic ground sumac

Preheat the oven to 350°F.

Heat 1 tablespoon of the oil in a large ovenproof frying pan over medium heat.

Add the leeks and shallots and cook, stirring frequently, for about 12 minutes, or until soft and golden brown. Add the chard, kale, and garlic and continue to cook, stirring, for 3 minutes, or until the greens have wilted. Stir in the lemon juice along with another 2 tablespoons of the olive oil. Continue to cook for a minute or so, stirring to blend completely.

Smooth out the top of the greens, then make four indentations in the top, each large enough to hold an egg. Carefully slip an egg into each indentation. Season with salt and pepper and transfer the pan to the preheated oven. Bake for about 15 minutes, or until the eggs are just set.

While the eggs are baking, place the remaining olive oil in a small saucepan. Add the tarragon, crushed red pepper, and sumac and place over medium heat. Season with salt and pepper and cook, stirring occasionally, for about 3 minutes, or until the oil is hot and fragrant.

Remove the pan from the oven. Drizzle the seasoned oil over the top and serve directly from the pan while hot.

Cauliflower Pancakes

Serves 4
Time required: About 25 minutes

Although these pancakes make a terrific breakfast or brunch dish, they are also a wonderful side dish for grilled meats, poultry, and/or fish. The turmeric adds great color as well as a slightly tannic yet sweet flavor.

- 1 pound organic cauliflower florets, including stems
- 1 small organic white onion, peeled and grated
- 1 teaspoon grated organic garlic
- ½ teaspoon organic ground turmeric
- 3 large eggs from pasture-raised chickens, at room temperature, lightly beaten
- Fine sea salt and freshly ground organic black pepper to taste
- ⅓ cup organic ghee from grass-fed animals
- ½ cup chopped organic scallion greens
- 1 cup full-fat organic sour cream from grass-fed cows (optional)

Preheat the oven to 200°F. Place a cookie sheet lined with parchment paper in the oven.

Using a handheld box grater, grate the cauliflower through the medium holes. Transfer the grated cauliflower in a large mixing bowl. Add the onion, garlic, and turmeric and toss to blend.

Add the eggs and season with sea salt and pepper, stirring to combine completely. Set aside for 10 minutes to allow the flavors to blossom.

Heat the ghee in a large frying pan over medium heat. Spoon in enough of the cauliflower mixture to make a flat cake about 3 inches in diameter. Continue making cakes without crowding the pan.

Using the back of a metal spatula, flatten the cakes slightly, but allow them to get no larger than 4 inches in diameter.

Fry for about 5 minutes, or until the bottom is golden brown and the pancakes have firmed enough to turn easily. Lower the heat if they are browning too quickly.

Using the spatula—a fish spatula is a great tool for this—carefully turn the pancakes and fry for an additional 4 minutes, or until cooked through and golden brown. If you flip them too quickly, they will fall apart.

As each one is cooked, place it on the cookie sheet in the oven and continue making cakes until all the batter has been used.

When ready to serve, place the pancakes on a platter, sprinkle with sea salt and scallion greens, and serve with sour cream on the side if desired.

APPETIZERS, SOUPS, SALADS, AND SMALL PLATES

Cauliflower Hummus

Serves 4 to 6

Time required: About 12 minutes

This is a light, tasty hummus. It is a wonderful dip for crudités but also makes a terrific sandwich on our Stone Age Bread (page 276). If you roast the cauliflower, the hummus will have a rich depth of flavor.

- 1 large head organic cauliflower, cut into florets and steamed until crisp-tender
- 4 cloves organic garlic, peeled, or more to taste
- ¼ cup organic tahini
- 1 teaspoon organic ground cumin
- Juice of 1 organic lemon, or more to taste
- Organic extra virgin olive oil to taste
- Fine sea salt to taste

Combine the cauliflower, garlic, tahini, and cumin in the bowl of a food processor fitted with a metal blade. Begin processing and, with the motor running, add the lemon juice a bit at a time until you get the amount of acidity that you like. Add just enough extra virgin olive oil to smooth out the mixture and add a bit of fruitiness. Season with salt to taste.

Scrape into a nonreactive container, cover, and refrigerate for up to one week.

Serve at room temperature with an assortment of raw vegetables.

VARIATION: If you want to add an elegant touch, sprinkle the top with fresh organic pomegranate seeds or with a mix of organic black and toasted white sesame seeds before serving.

Madras Pea Soup

Serves 6

Time required: About 40 minutes

The heat of the chili pepper and the savory East Indian spices make a great counterpoint to the sweet peas, cool yogurt, and aromatic herbs in this dish. Even when fresh peas are in season, use frozen organic peas for their beautiful color and consistent sweetness — fresh peas can be a bit dicey when it comes to color and starchiness. Served hot or cold, this is a filling soup that can, in larger portions, be used as a lunch or light supper entrée.

1 tablespoon organic coconut oil

¾ cup chopped organic white onion

1 tablespoon minced organic ginger

1 teaspoon minced organic garlic

2 teaspoons toasted organic cumin seeds, ground in a mortar and pestle

½ teaspoon organic ground coriander

½ teaspoon organic ground cinnamon

2 cups dried organic split peas

1 small organic carrot, peeled, trimmed, and chopped

1 organic serrano or jalapeño chili pepper, stemmed and chopped, or more to taste

3 cups Vegetable Stock (page 268) or organic canned vegetable broth

Fine sea salt to taste

Juice of 1 organic lemon

½ teaspoon organic garam masala

½ cup plain plain full-fat organic yogurt from grass-fed animals, plus more for garnish (optional)

Freshly ground organic black pepper to taste

1 cup frozen organic baby peas, thawed, drained, and patted dry (see Note)

1 tablespoon chopped organic cilantro

1 tablespoon chopped organic mint

6–8 sprigs organic cilantro or mint (optional)

Heat the oil in a large heavy-bottom saucepan over medium heat. Add the onion, ginger, and garlic and fry, stirring frequently, for about 5 minutes, or until the onions begin to take on some color. Stir in the cumin, coriander, and cinnamon and sauté for 1 minute. Add the split peas, carrot, chili pepper, and stock along with 3 cups of water and bring to a boil. Season with salt.

Lower the heat to a simmer and simmer for about 30 minutes, or until the peas are soft. If the mixture gets too thick, add stock or water ½ cup at a time.

Remove from the heat and stir in the lemon juice, garam masala, and ½ cup yogurt. Pour into a blender—in batches, if necessary—and process to a smooth puree.

Pour the puree into a clean saucepan. Place over medium heat and bring to a simmer, stirring frequently. Do not allow the soup to boil, or the yogurt might curdle. Add the pepper, taste, and adjust the seasoning if necessary.

Stir in the peas, chopped cilantro, and chopped mint. Pour into shallow soup bowls and, if desired, garnish the center with a dollop of yogurt and a cilantro or mint sprig.

NOTE: Do not allow the frozen peas to sit at room temperature for too long, or they will shrivel. It is a good idea to remove them from the freezer just a bit before needed, transfer to a strainer, and quickly defrost them under hot running water. The hot water thaws and warms them rapidly so that they can be patted dry and added to the soup without chilling it down.

VARIATION: This soup may also be served cold. After pureeing, cover and refrigerate for about 4 hours, or until well chilled. Stir in the peas, cilantro, and mint just before serving and, if desired, garnish as above. The soup may also be frozen.

Garlic Soup

Serves 4 to 6
Time required: About 40 minutes

A number of countries have a garlic soup all their own — Spain has sopa de ajo; in Portugal it's açorda à alentejana; in Italy it's the wondrous zuppa all'aglio; and the French have this one, known as Provençal aïgo bouïdo. It is a warming fall or winter filling-enough-to-be-a-main-course dish (when you add cheese and some of our Stone Age Bread — page 276), and the aroma coming from the kitchen will make you ravenous.

- 3 medium heads very fresh organic garlic, unpeeled
- 1 medium organic sweet onion, such as Vidalia, peeled and chopped
- 2 organic bay leaves
- 2 organic whole cloves
- 2 organic sage leaves
- 2 sprigs organic thyme
- Fine sea salt to taste

3 large organic egg yolks from pasture-raised chickens, at room temperature

¼ cup organic extra virgin olive oil

Freshly ground organic black pepper to taste (optional)

1 teaspoon chopped organic flat-leaf parsley

1 teaspoon chopped organic chives

Freshly grated organic Parmesan cheese for serving

Pour 2 quarts of water into a large saucepan and bring to a boil over high heat.

While the water is coming to a boil, using your fingers, push all the dry, loose skin from the garlic heads. Coarsely chop the heads, skin and all.

To the boiling water, add the chopped garlic along with the onion, bay leaves, cloves, sage leaves, and thyme sprigs. Add salt to taste and return to a low simmer. Simmer for about 25 minutes, or until the garlic is mushy.

While the broth is simmering, prepare the thickener. Place the egg yolks in a small mixing bowl. Using a whisk, beat the yolks until they are very light and quite thick. Whisking constantly, add the oil in a slow, steady stream, beating until the mixture reaches the consistency of mayonnaise. Cover and set aside until ready to use.

When the garlic is mushy, remove the broth from the heat and strain through a fine-mesh sieve, discarding the solids. Season the broth with salt and pepper.

Return the strained liquid to the saucepan and bring to a boil over medium heat.

Meanwhile, scrape the thickener into a soup tureen or large serving bowl. Once the broth has come to a boil, remove it from the heat and, whisking the thickener constantly, slowly pour about a cup of the hot broth into the thickener; then pour in the remaining broth. Sprinkle chopped parsley and chives over the top. Serve individual portions with a healthy dose of grated Parmesan over the top.

Chicken Caesar Salad

Serves 4
Time required: About 35 minutes

This salad contains what looks like a lot of ingredients, but they're not difficult to pull together. The dressing and the chicken can be made early in the day and the kale roasted an hour or so ahead of serving. Then it's 1-2-3 to put it all together for this elegant version of a Caesar salad.

3 large organic egg yolks from pasture-raised chickens, at room temperature

1 tablespoon organic whole-grain mustard

1 teaspoon organic Dijon mustard

1 teaspoon organic anchovy paste

1 teaspoon Roasted Garlic (pages 319–20)

1 tablespoon organic cider vinegar

½ cup organic extra virgin olive oil, divided

Fine sea salt and freshly ground organic black pepper to taste

4 boneless, skinless organic chicken breasts from pasture-raised chickens, about 6 ounces each

⅓ cup finely grated organic Parmesan cheese

8 organic kale leaves, trimmed of their tough stalks

2 heads organic baby romaine lettuce, well washed and separated into leaves

3 cups organic baby spinach leaves

1 cup shredded organic brussels sprouts

½ cup thinly sliced organic radishes

½ cup sliced raw unsalted organic almonds, toasted

Combine the egg yolks, mustards, anchovy paste, garlic, and vinegar in a small mixing bowl. Slowly pour in ¼ cup of the olive oil, whisking to emulsify. Season with salt and pepper and set aside.

Preheat the oven to 300°F. Line a baking sheet with parchment paper and set aside.

Preheat an outdoor grill or preheat a stovetop grill pan over high heat.

Trim the chicken of any membrane or sinew. Generously rub all sides with about 2 tablespoons of the remaining olive oil and season with salt and pepper.

Place the chicken breasts on the hot grill or pan and cook, turning frequently, for about 10 minutes, or until just cooked through and the temperature on an instant-read thermometer reaches 155°F. Remove from the heat and set aside. The chicken will continue to cook as it rests and should reach at least 160°F.

While the chicken is cooking, prepare the kale. Combine the remaining olive oil with the Parmesan cheese and salt and pepper to taste in a small bowl, whisking to blend completely. Using a pastry brush, coat both sides of the kale leaves with the mixture.

Place the seasoned kale leaves on the prepared baking sheet in the preheated oven and roast for about 20 minutes, or until the kale is lightly browned and crisp. Remove from the oven and set aside.

When ready to serve, cut the chicken crosswise into thin slices. Set aside.

Combine the romaine, spinach, brussels sprouts, radishes, and almonds in a large mixing bowl. Add the sliced chicken along with about half the mustard dressing and toss to combine.

Place equal portions of the salad on each of four luncheon plates. Place an equal portion of roasted kale on top of each serving.

Serve immediately with the remaining dressing on the side.

Chicory Salad with Tahini Dressing

Serves 4

Time required: About 15 minutes

This is an invigorating salad, combining the bitterness of the greens, the warmth of the nuts, and the creaminess of the dressing. In choosing your greens, try to find some purple, some green, and some speckled chicories to make the salad visually exciting, too.

3/4 pound mixed organic chicories, such as frisée, Belgian endive, radicchio, or other bitter leafy greens

½ cup coarsely chopped unsalted organic walnuts, toasted

Tahini Dressing to taste (below)

About ¼ cup organic pomegranate seeds (optional)

Combine the greens and walnuts in a large salad bowl. Add just enough dressing to lightly coat and toss to blend well.

Serve immediately with pomegranate seeds strewn over the top, if desired.

Tahini Dressing

Makes about 6 tablespoons
Time required: About 15 minutes

2 tablespoons organic tahini

½ teaspoon minced organic garlic

Zest and juice of ½ small organic orange

3 tablespoons organic extra virgin olive oil

Fine sea salt and freshly ground organic black pepper to taste

Combine the tahini with the garlic and orange zest and juice in a small mixing bowl. Slowly whisk in the olive oil and season with salt and pepper.

If the dressing seems too thick or grainy, add cool water a tablespoon at a time until the desired consistency is reached. The dressing should resemble thick cream.

Sesame Beef Kebabs with Avocado Dipping Sauce

Makes 28 pieces
Time required: About 15 minutes, plus 1 hour for soaking skewers

This would be a fun appetizer or snack for a summer grilling party because you could get everything together and then let your guests grill their own kebabs.

The dipping sauce adds a bit of zest, but the kebabs are great on their own, too.

> 2 organic New York strip or rib-eye steaks from grass-fed cows, about 1 pound each, trimmed of all fat
>
> Fine sea salt and freshly cracked organic black pepper to taste
>
> 1 cup organic sesame seeds
>
> 1 cup organic avocado oil
>
> 1 recipe Avocado Dipping Sauce (below; optional)

Place twenty-eight 8-inch bamboo skewers in cold water and let soak for at least 1 hour. Drain well, but do not allow the skewers to dry out.

Using a sharp knife, trim a thin edge off the sides of each steak to make two neat rectangles, each about 7 inches long by 4 inches wide by 1 inch thick. Cut each steak crosswise into 7 pieces, each about 4 inches long and 1 inch wide.

Place the 14 pieces of meat alongside one another with the length facing away from you. Weave two bamboo skewers up through each piece of meat so that when the strip is cut in half down the middle after cooking you will have two skewers of beef of equal size. (The skewers may be assembled up to this point and stored, covered, and refrigerated, for up to 24 hours or frozen for up to three months.)

When ready to cook, place the sesame seeds on a clean flat surface. Season the meat with salt and pepper, then roll each skewer in sesame seeds to completely cover.

Pour the oil into a nonstick griddle or stovetop grill pan set over medium-high heat. When the oil is shimmering, place the skewers in the hot oil and sear, turning occasionally, for about 2 minutes, or until the meat is nicely browned but still rare in the center.

Transfer the skewers to a cutting board and cut each one in half to make two smaller skewers of equal size. Lay the skewers out on a serving platter cut side up to show the rareness of the meat.

Serve immediately with the dipping sauce on the side if desired.

Avocado Dipping Sauce

Makes about 1 cup
Time required: About 15 minutes

  1 large ripe organic avocado, peeled and pitted

  ⅓ cup plain full-fat organic yogurt from grass-fed animals

  2 tablespoons grated organic red onion

  1 teaspoon grated organic ginger

  Fine sea salt and freshly ground organic black pepper to taste

  Freshly grated organic green chili pepper to taste (optional)

Place the avocado, yogurt, onion, and ginger in the bowl of a food processor fitted with a metal blade and process until very smooth. Taste and season with salt and pepper and, if desired, freshly grated chili pepper.

Grilled Clams with Citrus-Herb Sauce

Serves 4 to 6
Time required: About 15 minutes

This is a perfect summer appetizer, cocktail tidbit, or snack. Grilling clams is quick and easy to do while chatting with guests. When the clams are topped with a light, refreshing herb sauce, there is nothing more elegant or good for you. The sauce is also terrific on grilled fish, poultry, or meat.

3 dozen wild clams, well scrubbed (see Note)

Citrus-Herb Sauce to taste (below)

Preheat an outdoor grill to high.

Place the clams on the grill with the flatter side up. This will help hold the juices in the rounder side as the clams open from the heat. Grill for about 4 minutes, or until the clams open.

As they open, remove the clams from the grill, dollop with a bit of the sauce, and eat them hot, straight from the shell.

NOTE: Fresh wild clams need to be soaked in salt water, preferably the same water they came from, to allow them to expunge the sand from their shells.

Citrus-Herb Sauce

Makes about 2 cups

2 cups chopped organic flat-leaf parsley

½ cup chopped organic leeks, including some green parts

¼ cup chopped organic cilantro

2 tablespoons chopped organic oregano

1 tablespoon chopped organic garlic

½ teaspoon freshly grated organic orange zest

Juice and zest of 1 organic lemon

1 cup organic extra virgin olive oil

¼ cup organic champagne vinegar

Fine sea salt to taste

Combine the parsley, leeks, cilantro, oregano, garlic, and orange zest in the bowl of a food processor fitted with a metal blade and pulse until just minced. Add the lemon juice and zest and process to just incorporate. Scrape the mixture into a nonreactive container. Stir in the oil and vinegar. Season with salt, cover, and refrigerate until ready to use.

ENTRÉES

Lamb with Mustard Sauce

Serves 4

Time required: About 30 minutes

This is a very easy "company's coming" recipe. The spices accent the rich, juicy lamb beautifully. It is easy to double or triple the spices to coat as many lamb racks as you need.

> 3 tablespoons organic whole-grain mustard
>
> 1¼ teaspoons organic ground turmeric
>
> 1 teaspoon organic garam masala
>
> ½ teaspoon organic chili powder
>
> 2 tablespoons organic coconut oil
>
> Fine sea salt to taste
>
> 1 (8-rib) rack organic grass-fed lamb, about 1½ pounds

Preheat the oven to 425°F.

Combine the mustard, turmeric, garam masala, chili powder, and coconut oil in a small bowl, stirring to blend completely. Season with salt.

Generously rub the mustard mixture over the lamb. Place the coated meat in a roasting pan and roast for about 20 minutes, or until an instant-read thermometer inserted into the thickest part reads 140°F (which will yield rare meat if served immediately).

Place the rack on a cutting board and let rest for about 10 minutes, or until the thermometer registers 150°F for medium rare.

Using a chef's knife, cut through each rack along the bone and serve 2 chops per person.

Deviled Cornish Game Hens

Serves 4 to 6
Time required: About 25 minutes

Although this recipe calls for game hens, it could easily be prepared with chicken, turkey, pork, or seafood. The sauce would also be very tasty served with cauliflower steaks or grilled vegetables.

- 1 tablespoon organic tamarind paste dissolved in 2 tablespoons warm water
- 2 fresh organic red or green hot chili peppers, stemmed and seeded, or more to taste
- 1 cup unsweetened organic coconut milk
- ¼ cup minced organic yellow onion
- 1 tablespoon minced organic garlic
- Fine sea salt to taste
- 3 whole organic pasture-raised Cornish game hens, cleaned and split in half lengthwise
- Juice of 1 organic lemon

Preheat an outdoor grill to high.

Strain the tamarind through a fine-mesh sieve, pressing on the solids to extract all the liquid. You should have around 1 tablespoon. Discard the solids. In the bowl of a food processor, combine the tamarind liquid with the chili peppers, coconut milk, onion, and garlic and process until smooth. Season with salt to taste.

Generously rub the hens with lemon juice. Place on the preheated grill and grill each side for 2 minutes. Remove from the grill and set aside. Keep the grill hot.

Using the flat side of a cleaver or a heavy-bottom frying pan, pound each hen half to flatten it slightly.

Place the flattened hens, skin side down, in a large frying pan. Add the tamarind mixture and place over medium heat. Bring to a boil, then lower the heat and simmer for 6 minutes.

Immediately remove the hens from the sauce and return to the hot grill. Grill, skin side down, for 4 minutes, or until crisp. Remove from the grill and serve immediately with or without the sauce from the pan.

Almost Tandoori Chicken

Serves 4 to 6
Time required: About 1 hour, plus 24 hours for marinating

This is an unusual take on classic oven-roasted chicken. In case you are unfamiliar with it, a tandoor is a traditional Indian clay oven (it's also used in other Asian cuisines) heated with wood or charcoal. Temperatures in the oven are maintained at 450°F to 500°F. But if you don't have a tandoor, we find that a backyard grill can also turn out an absolutely delicious roast chicken. It may not look quite as glorious as a tandoor-burnished traditional Indian chicken, but it is still very tasty. Just a hint of spice permeates the extremely tender, moist meat.

2½ cups plain full-fat organic yogurt from grass-fed animals

2 tablespoons freshly squeezed organic lime juice

½–1 organic hot red chili pepper, seeded and chopped

¾ cup chopped organic yellow onion

1 tablespoon minced fresh organic ginger

1 teaspoon minced fresh organic garlic

1 tablespoon organic paprika

2 teaspoons organic garam masala

1 teaspoon organic ground turmeric

1 whole organic pasture-raised roasting chicken, about 3½–4 pounds

Combine the yogurt and lime juice in the bowl of a food processor fitted with a metal blade and process to just combine. Add the chili pepper, onion, ginger, and garlic and process to blend. Add the paprika, garam masala, and turmeric and process until almost smooth.

Cut small slits in the skin of the chicken so it will absorb the marinade, then place it in a large resealable plastic bag. Add the yogurt mixture, seal, and toss to cover well. Place in the refrigerator and allow to marinate for 24 hours (but no longer), turning the bag from time to time to ensure that the entire chicken is tenderized by the marinade.

About 30 minutes before you are ready to roast, preheat your oven to 500°F or make a very hot charcoal fire on one side of an outdoor grill—you will want the temperature to reach 500°F before you cook the chicken.

Remove the chicken from the plastic bag and turn it so that excess marinade drips out of the cavity. Discard the marinade. Place the chicken on a rack in a roasting pan or on the grill rack on the far opposite side of the fire. Cover and begin roasting, turning the chicken occasionally to ensure that it is cooking evenly. Add charcoal as necessary to the grill to maintain the hot fire. In the oven, this should take no more than 40 minutes; on the grill, it can take about 2 hours for the chicken to be perfectly cooked throughout.

Remove from the oven or grill and let rest for about 15 minutes before cutting into pieces.

Whole Roasted Striped Bass

Serves 6
Time required: About 40 minutes

You can adapt this recipe to any whole firm fish, or, if you prefer, you can use nice thick fillets of any sweet, firm-fleshed wild fish, such as salmon or halibut. We find that roasting whole fish at a high temperature seals in its juices so it remains extremely moist.

> 2 whole wild striped bass, 3 pounds each, gutted and cleaned
>
> 2 unpeeled organic lemons, well washed and thinly sliced crosswise
>
> 10 sprigs organic tarragon, plus more for garnish if desired
>
> 10 sprigs organic flat-leaf parsley, plus more for garnish if desired
>
> 3 tablespoons organic extra virgin olive oil
>
> 2 tablespoons freshly squeezed organic lemon juice
>
> Fine sea salt and freshly ground organic black pepper to taste
>
> 2 large organic fennel bulbs, thinly sliced crosswise
>
> 3 cups (about 2 pounds) peeled and sliced organic shallots, blanched
>
> ½ cup organic dry white wine

Preheat the oven to 450°F.

Rinse the fish and pat dry, both inside and out.

Layer half the lemon slices in the cavity of one of the fish. Place about 5 sprigs each of tarragon and parsley on top of the lemons. Repeat with the other fish.

Combine the olive oil and lemon juice in a small bowl. Using your hands, generously coat both fish with the oil mixture. Season both sides with salt and pepper.

Combine the fennel and shallots in a shallow roasting pan large enough to hold both fish. Season with salt and pepper and smooth the vegetables out to an even layer. Pour the wine into the pan, then place the fish on top of the vegetables.

Place the pan in the preheated oven and roast, turning the vegetables occasionally, for about 25 minutes, or until the vegetables are tender and an instant-read thermometer inserted into the thickest part of the fish reads 135°F.

Remove the pan from the oven and allow the fish to rest for 5 minutes.

Using two spatulas, carefully lift each fish from the roasting pan onto a serving platter. Spoon the fennel-shallot mixture around each fish and, if desired, garnish with chopped tarragon or parsley and fresh lemon slices.

Salmon with Green Sauce

Serves 4
Time required: About 15 minutes

This is such an easy recipe that you can pull it together in a few minutes. It is perfect for a weekday meal or even a celebratory dinner, because it looks so pretty on the plate.

2 bunches organic arugula (or spinach or any other bitter green), well washed

⅓ cup organic unsalted butter from grass-fed cows

Fine sea salt and and freshly ground organic black pepper to taste

1 tablespoon organic coconut oil

4 skinless wild salmon fillets, 6 ounces each

Organic ground cumin for dusting

Place the arugula in boiling water for about 30 seconds to blanch. Drain well and pat dry.

Transfer the blanched greens to a blender (or food processor fitted with a metal blade) and process to a saucelike consistency, adding a bit of warm water as needed to smooth out.

Scrape the puree into a small saucepan, add the butter, salt, and pepper, and set over low heat to warm through. Remove from the heat and keep warm. (The puree can be made in advance and reheated in a double boiler.)

Heat the coconut oil in a large frying pan over high heat.

Season the salmon with salt and pepper and dust both sides with cumin. Place in the hot pan and sear, turning once, for about 6 minutes, or until nicely colored on the exterior and rare in the center.

Place a salmon fillet in the center of each of four serving plates and drizzle the green puree around the edge. Serve immediately.

Whole Roasted Salmon with Sunchokes and Leeks

Serves 6

Time required: About 30 minutes

If you can't get a whole six-pound salmon, don't hesitate to use a smaller fish or just roast one side of a larger salmon. This recipe can also be prepared with striped bass or any other slightly fatty fish and served hot or at room temperature. It is a lovely dish for guests, filling them with the prebiotic goodness of the sunchokes and leeks.

- 1½ pounds small organic sunchokes, scrubbed
- 3 branches organic rosemary, 5 inches each, or other herb of choice
- 1 unpeeled organic lemon, sliced crosswise
- 1 whole wild salmon, about 6 pounds, gutted and cleaned, head and tail left on, rinsed and patted dry
- Fine sea salt and freshly ground organic black pepper to taste
- 1 tablespoon organic coconut oil
- 6 organic leeks, including a trace of the green parts, trimmed, well washed, and sliced lengthwise
- 1 teaspoon fresh organic rosemary leaves
- Organic lemon wedges for garnish (optional)
- Organic watercress sprigs for garnish (optional)

Bring a large pot of salted water to a boil over high heat. Add the sunchokes, lower the heat, and simmer for about 5 minutes, or until just slightly cooked. Drain and pat dry. Set aside.

Preheat the oven to 375°F.

Place the rosemary branches and lemon slices in the cavity of the fish. Season with salt and pepper. Using a pastry brush, lightly coat the top of the salmon with coconut oil.

Place the reserved sunchokes and the leeks in a roasting pan large enough to hold the salmon. Sprinkle the vegetables with the rosemary leaves and season with salt and pepper. Lay the salmon on top of the vegetables.

Place in the preheated oven and roast for about 15 minutes per inch of thickness of the fish, or until an instant-read thermometer reads 135°F when inserted into the thickest part of the salmon.

Remove the pan from the oven and allow the fish to rest for 10 minutes.

Serve the salmon and vegetables garnished with lemon wedges and watercress, if desired.

Vegetable Lasagna

Serves 4 to 8
Time required: About 1½ hours

We like this lasagna not only with zucchini instead of pasta but also with slices of grilled eggplant instead of pasta. It is a rich meal, and the pasta and meat won't be missed at all. It's also a great dish to carry to parties, potlucks, or almost any gathering. Guests will be grateful for the introduction of this lighter, more healthful version of the beloved Italian classic.

3½ pounds organic zucchini

Fine sea salt to taste

2 tablespoons organic extra virgin olive oil

1 cup finely diced organic yellow onion

1 tablespoon smashed organic garlic

1 can (28 ounces) plus 1 cup organic crushed tomatoes

1 tablespoon organic dried basil

2 teaspoons organic dried oregano

¼ teaspoon organic crushed red pepper flakes

Freshly ground organic black pepper to taste

5½ cups shredded organic full-fat mozzarella cheese from grass-fed animals, divided

2 cups Ricotta Cheese (page 275)

2 cups grated organic Parmesan cheese, divided

1 large organic egg from pasture-raised chickens, at room temperature

Preheat the oven to 375°F.

Line two baking sheets with parchment paper. Set aside.

Using a handheld vegetable slicer or a mandolin, cut the zucchini lengthwise into ¼-inch-thick slices. Lay the slices in a single layer on the prepared baking sheets. Sprinkle the slices with salt and set aside for 10 minutes. This will draw some of the moisture out of the vegetables and prevent the lasagna from becoming runny.

After 10 minutes, use a paper towel to gently pat the zucchini dry.

Transfer the baking sheets to the preheated oven and roast for about 12 minutes, or until the zucchini slices are beginning to color around the edges. Remove from the oven and set aside.

Heat the olive oil in a large saucepan over medium heat. Add the onion and garlic and cook, stirring frequently, for about 4 minutes, or just until the vegetables are starting to soften. Add the tomatoes along with the basil, oregano, and red pepper flakes. Season with salt and pepper and bring to a simmer. Cook, stirring occasionally, for about 15 minutes, or until the sauce has thickened slightly. Taste and, if necessary, season with additional salt and pepper.

Combine 2 cups of the mozzarella with the Ricotta Cheese and 1 cup of the Parmesan in the bowl of a food processor fitted with a metal blade. Add the egg and season with salt and pepper. Pulse until the mixture is completely smooth.

Spoon about 1 cup of the tomato mixture on the bottom of a 12 × 16-inch baking pan. Lay about one-fourth of the zucchini slices on top, followed by about 1 cup of the cheese mixture, taking care that it covers the zucchini completely. Top with a layer of about 1 cup mozzarella and about ¼ cup Parmesan. Repeat the layering two more times. Then add a layer of zucchini slices followed by the remaining ½ cup of mozzarella. Finish with the remaining ¼ cup of Parmesan.

Place the lasagna in the preheated oven and bake for 30 minutes. Increase the oven temperature to 500°F and continue to bake for about 5 minutes, or until the cheese is golden brown and the lasagna is very hot and bubbling.

Remove from the oven and set on a wire rack to settle for about 15 minutes before cutting and serving.

Grilled Cauliflower and Broccoli Steaks with Eggplant

Serves 4

Time required: About 45 minutes

Vegetable steaks look great on the plate and serve as a marvelous introduction to healthful eating. If you don't have time to make the eggplant or the dressing, just grill the "steaks" and drizzle with a vinaigrette or some extra virgin olive oil and balsamic vinegar.

1 organic globe eggplant (about 2 pounds), trimmed

¾ cup organic extra virgin olive oil, plus more for coating grill pan

Fine sea salt to taste

Organic cayenne pepper to taste

1 large head organic cauliflower, trimmed and cut lengthwise into 1-inch-thick slices

1 large head organic broccoli, trimmed and cut into 4 equal pieces

¼ cup organic oregano leaves

1 tablespoon mashed Roasted Garlic (see Note)

1 tablespoon organic fennel seeds

Organic cracked black pepper to taste

Tahini Dressing to taste (page 300)

Organic ground sumac for garnish (optional)

Preheat an outdoor grill or a stovetop grill pan over high heat.

Line two large baking pans with parchment. Set aside.

Cut the eggplant in half lengthwise and, using about ¼ cup of the olive oil, generously oil each half. Place the eggplant cut side down on the grill or grill pan. Grill, turning occasionally, for about 30 minutes, or until the flesh is crinkled and golden brown and the skin has blackened and charred.

Remove the eggplant from the heat and slip the skin off the flesh. Season with the salt and cayenne pepper and stir, adding just enough olive oil to create a soft, smooth puree. Set aside but keep warm.

While the eggplant is cooking, prepare the cauliflower and broccoli.

Pour the remaining olive oil in a small bowl. Add the oregano, Roasted Garlic, and fennel seeds. Season with salt and cracked pepper. Using a pastry brush, generously coat both sides of the cauliflower and broccoli with the seasoned oil. Place the vegetables on the lined baking sheets to marinate for a few minutes.

When the eggplant comes off the grill, carefully transfer the vegetable steaks to the grill. Grill, turning once, for about 6 minutes, or until the steaks are just barely tender.

Spoon an equal portion of the eggplant into the center of each of four dinner plates. Layer a cauliflower steak onto the eggplant and place a broccoli steak at its side. Drizzle with Tahini Dressing and garnish with a sprinkle of ground sumac if desired.

Serve immediately.

NOTE: To make Roasted Garlic, preheat the oven to 350°F. Lightly coat either unpeeled whole heads of organic garlic or peeled individual cloves with organic extra virgin olive oil, wrap in aluminum foil, and place on a baking pan in the preheated oven. If you're serving whole heads on a platter with grilled meats, make a nice, neat slice off the top before roasting. Whole heads will take about 25 minutes to become soft and aromatic; individual cloves will take about 12 minutes.

To make roasted garlic puree, roast whole heads as directed above and, when they're soft and aromatic, cut off the tops and squeeze out the lush, soft flesh. One large head will usually yield about 2 tablespoons of puree. Roasted garlic is rich, deeply flavorful, and not at all pungent.

SIDES

Jicama Slaw
———

Serves 4 to 6
Time required: About 20 minutes

This terrific prebiotic side dish goes splendidly with grilled wild fish, chicken, or pork, particularly if it has a little spice added. It is a refreshing and healthful substitute for regular coleslaw and would be most welcome at a summertime barbecue or picnic.

Juice of 2 small organic oranges

Juice of 1 organic lime

2 cloves organic garlic, peeled

1 bunch organic cilantro leaves

¼ cup organic extra virgin olive oil

3 small organic jicama, peeled and cut into julienne strips

1 organic red onion, peeled and cut into julienne strips

1 bunch organic mint leaves, cut into slivers

1 bunch organic scallions, thinly sliced diagonally

Combine the citrus juices, garlic, cilantro, and olive oil in a blender and process until almost smooth. Set aside until ready to use.

Place the jicama, onions, mint, and scallions in a large salad bowl. Add enough of the dressing to lightly coat the salad.

Serve immediately.

Sautéed Asparagus

Serves 4 to 6
Time required: About 10 minutes

Asparagus prepared in this way has a bit more interesting flavor than when steamed and served with lemon. This piquant mixture works well as an accompaniment to almost any meat, poultry, or game and as a luncheon course topped with poached or scrambled eggs.

- 2 tablespoons organic ghee from grass-fed animals
- 2 small organic shallots, peeled and thinly sliced
- 2 bunches organic green asparagus, trimmed and cut in half
- 2 sprigs organic thyme leaves
- 1 pickled chili pepper, seeded and minced
- Fine sea salt and freshly ground organic white pepper to taste
- ½ tablespoon organic sherry vinegar

Heat the ghee in a large sauté pan over medium heat. Add the shallots and cook, stirring frequently, for 3 minutes, or until translucent. Add the asparagus, thyme, and chili pepper. Season with salt and pepper and cook, tossing and stirring frequently, for about 7 minutes, or until the asparagus is just crisp-tender.

About a minute before the asparagus is ready, deglaze the pan with the sherry vinegar. Toss and remove from the heat.

Serve immediately.

Zucchini and Parsnip Noodles with Celery Root in Broccoli Sauce

Serves 4
Time required: About 20 minutes

Although a vegetable-noodle maker, or spiralizer, is now a fixture in many kitchens, some supermarkets also sell precut noodles made from zucchini, carrots, beets, and other firm vegetables. We like to make our own because we can control the quality and freshness of the vegetables, but any way you cut them, vegetable noodles make a delicious side dish or even a main course.

8 cups (about 1 pound) organic broccoli florets

½ cup finely grated organic Parmesan cheese, plus more
for sprinkling

⅓ cup unsalted raw organic cashews

Fine sea salt to taste

¼ cup organic extra virgin olive oil, plus more for drizzling

2 cloves organic garlic, peeled and thinly sliced

1 organic hot red chili pepper, trimmed, seeded, and
finely chopped, or more to taste

1 tablespoon freshly grated organic lemon zest

1½ pounds organic zucchini noodles

½ pound organic parsnip noodles

½ pound organic celery root, shredded

Combine the broccoli, ½ cup Parmesan, cashews, and salt in the bowl of a food processor fitted with a metal blade. Process until fine crumbs form.

Heat ¼ cup oil in a large frying pan over medium heat. Add the garlic and chili pepper and sauté, stirring frequently, for about 2 minutes, or until the garlic is soft but not colored. Add the broccoli mixture along with the lemon zest and continue to cook, stirring, for about 10 minutes, or until the mixture is browning and very fragrant.

Add the zucchini, parsnip, and celery root and cook, tossing, for about 3 minutes, or until the noodles are coated with the sauce and warmed through.

Remove from the heat and serve drizzled with more olive oil and sprinkled with Parmesan cheese.

Sunchoke Gratin

Serves 4

Time required: About 35 minutes

When made into a gratin, sunchokes become slightly sweet. We add a healthy dose of black pepper to offset the sweetness and accent the mellowness of the finished dish. Like many of the side dishes in this chapter, this gratin can also work as a main course for lunch or a light supper.

- 2 tablespoons organic unsalted butter from grass-fed cows
- 1 tablespoon organic avocado oil
- 1 large organic white onion, peeled and cut lengthwise into thin wedges
- 1 pound organic sunchokes, peeled and cut crosswise into ⅛-inch-thick slices
- 1 tablespoon chopped organic thyme leaves
- Fine sea salt and freshly ground organic black pepper to taste
- ¼ cup organic crème fraîche from grass-fed cows
- 2 ounces grated organic Cheddar cheese from grass-fed cows

Combine the butter and oil in a large ovenproof frying pan over medium heat. Add the onion and cook, stirring frequently, for about 10 minutes, or until the onion is soft and beginning to color.

Add the sunchokes and thyme and generously season with salt and pepper. Add ½ cup water and bring to a simmer. Lower the heat, cover, and cook for about 20 minutes, or until the sunchokes are very tender. Uncover and simmer until the pan juices are reduced to a thick glaze, adding water a tablespoon at a time if necessary.

Preheat the broiler.

Dollop the crème fraîche over the top of the sunchokes and spread it into an even layer. Sprinkle the cheese over the top and immediately transfer to the broiler.

Broil for about 4 minutes, or until the top is golden brown and the edges are bubbling.

Remove from the broiler and serve.

Leeks and Swiss Chard with Coconut Milk

Serves 4
Time required: About 20 minutes

The combination of leeks and chard seems a bit bland, but once you heat things up with the garlic and curry and add the richness of the coconut milk, you have a dish that is anything but bland. You can use kale or another green in place of the chard, but try not to use a very bitter green because it will overpower the sweetness of the leeks.

5 organic leeks, including white and tender green parts, trimmed and well washed

2 tablespoons organic ghee from grass-fed cows

2 cloves organic garlic, peeled and sliced

½ pound organic Swiss chard leaves, trimmed of tough stalks and cut crosswise into ribbons

1 teaspoon organic hot curry powder

¼ teaspoon organic ground turmeric

Fine sea salt to taste

1⅔ cups organic unsweetened coconut milk

¼ cup chopped toasted organic unsalted nuts, such as a mix of almonds, walnuts, cashews, and macadamia nuts

Cut the leeks crosswise into ½-inch-thick diagonal slices.

Heat the ghee in a large frying pan over medium-low heat. Add the garlic and fry, stirring frequently, for a couple of minutes, or just until it softens but hasn't taken on any color.

Add the leeks along with the chard and continue to cook, stirring frequently, for about 5 minutes, or until the vegetables begin to soften. Add the curry powder and turmeric and season with salt. Cook, stirring, for another 3 minutes, or until the leeks are tender.

Add the coconut milk and bring to a simmer. Simmer for about 4 minutes, or just until the mixture begins to bubble.

Remove from the heat, scrape into a serving bowl, and sprinkle with chopped nuts.

Serve immediately.

Broccoli with Shallots and Red Pepper

Serves 4

Time required: About 15 minutes

It is important not to overcook the broccoli in this simple but tasty recipe, because you want it to be slightly crisp and not one bit wilted. You can also add some crushed red pepper flakes if you are in the mood for some spice.

8 cups (about 1 pound) organic broccoli florets

2 tablespoons organic coconut oil

2 organic shallots, peeled and cut crosswise into thin slices

1 small organic red bell pepper, trimmed, seeded, deveined, and finely diced

1 teaspoon minced organic garlic

Fine sea salt and freshly ground organic black pepper to taste

Place the broccoli in the basket of a steamer with an inch or so of water in the bottom. Make sure the steamer basket does not touch the water. Cover, place over high heat, and bring the water to a boil. Steam the broccoli for 2 minutes, then immediately remove the steamer basket from the heat and set aside.

Heat the oil in a large frying pan over medium heat. Add the shallots, bell pepper, and garlic and fry, stirring frequently, for about 5 minutes, or until the vegetables begin to soften. Add the steamed broccoli, season with salt and pepper, and cook, stirring, for another minute or two.

Transfer to a serving bowl and serve immediately.

Dandelion Greens with Onions

Serves 4

Time required: About 30 minutes

Dandelion greens are best in the spring, when they are small, young, tender, and not as bitter as the older greens will be. They are an excellent source of vitamins and prebiotics and should be eaten far more often than they are. You can pick your own, but you must make sure they are pristine, without having come into contact with toxic sprays or animal contaminants.

> 2 pounds organic dandelion greens, tough stems removed, chopped
>
> ¼ cup plus 1 tablespoon organic extra virgin olive oil
>
> 1 large organic onion, peeled and cut crosswise into thin rings
>
> 1 cup chopped organic shallots
>
> 1 tablespoon chopped organic garlic
>
> ¾ cup chopped mixed organic herbs, such as parsley, cilantro, chives, and basil
>
> Fine sea salt to taste
>
> Juice of 1 organic lemon

Bring a large pot of salted water to a boil over high heat. Add the chopped dandelion greens and boil for about 3 minutes, or just until tender.

Drain the greens through a fine-mesh strainer, then transfer to a large clean kitchen towel. Twist the towel together and wring the greens as dry as you can. Set aside.

Place ¼ cup of the oil in a large frying pan over medium-high heat. When the oil is very hot but not shimmering, add the sliced onion. Stir to break the onions apart and coat all the pieces with the oil. Cook, stirring occasionally, for about 5 minutes, or until the onions begin to brown. Lower the heat to medium-low and continue to cook, stirring occasionally, for about 15 minutes, or until the onions are golden brown and quite crisp.

Using a slotted spoon, transfer the onions to a double layer of paper towels to drain. Season with salt.

Place the remaining tablespoon of oil in a large saucepan. Add the shallots and garlic and cook, stirring frequently, for about 5 minutes, or until just starting to color slightly.

Add the reserved greens along with the chopped herbs and cook, stirring, to heat through. Taste and, if necessary, season with salt.

Remove from the heat and transfer to a serving dish. Drizzle with lemon juice and sprinkle the crisp onions over the top.

Serve immediately.

DESSERTS

Favorite Chocolate Cake

Makes one 9-inch cake
Time required: About 1¼ hours, plus 4 or more hours for chilling

Not only is this cake flourless, it is also sugarless! But it is delicious, too. It does have to chill before cutting, so it is best made the day before you need to serve it. It travels well and would make a great contribution to a bake sale, community event, or potluck dinner.

> 5 large organic eggs from pasture-raised chickens, separated, at room temperature
>
> Pinch of fine sea salt
>
> 9 ounces organic dark chocolate, at least 80% cacao
>
> ⅔ cup unsalted organic butter from grass-fed cows
>
> 2 teaspoons pure organic vanilla extract
>
> Organic cocoa powder for dusting

Preheat the oven to 325°F.

Generously butter the interior of a 9-inch round springform pan. Cut a parchment circle to fit the bottom of the pan and generously butter it as well.

Place the egg whites in the bowl of an electric mixer fitted with a whisk attachment. Add the salt and beat on low speed until stiff peaks form. Set aside.

Place the chocolate and butter in the top half of a double boiler over boiling water and heat, stirring frequently, for about 4 minutes, or until the chocolate and butter have melted and combined. Scrape the mixture into a large mixing bowl and, using a whisk, beat the egg yolks into the chocolate mixture one at a time. Beat in the vanilla.

Gently fold in the egg whites, a bit at a time, until no white streaks remain.

Pour the batter into the prepared pan and transfer to the preheated oven. Bake for about an hour, or until the cake jiggles in the center but the outer edges are firm.

Remove from the oven and set on a wire rack to cool. When cool, transfer to the refrigerator to set for at least 4 hours or overnight.

When ready to serve, unmold from the springform pan, then pull off and discard the parchment paper.

Place the cocoa powder in a fine-mesh sieve and gently tap to dust the top of the cake with cocoa.

Cut into slices and serve.

Chocolate Chip Cookies

Makes about 2 dozen
Time required: About 20 minutes

We love the combination of almond flavors and chocolate in these cookies. It is important that you use chocolate chips with at least 80% cacao. And if you toast the almonds, the cookies will have an even deeper almond flavor. These make a great introduction to the Brain Wash diet.

1¼ cups organic almond flour

¼ cup granulated organic stevia

¼ teaspoon baking soda

¼ cup organic coconut oil

2 teaspoons pure organic vanilla extract

½ cup organic dark chocolate chips, at least 80% cacao

½ cup chopped raw unsalted organic almonds or walnuts

Preheat the oven to 350°F.

Line two baking sheets with nonstick silicone liners or parchment paper.

Combine the almond flour, stevia, and baking soda in a medium mixing bowl. Stir in the coconut oil and vanilla. When well combined, stir in the chocolate chips and nuts.

Drop the dough by the heaping teaspoonfuls onto the prepared baking sheets. Transfer to the preheated oven and bake for about 9 minutes, or until set and golden around the edges.

Remove from the oven and, using a spatula, transfer to wire racks to cool.

Store in an airtight container at room temperature for no more than five days.

Almond-Coconut Biscotti

Makes 8 to 10
Time required: 1 hour, plus 12 hours for resting if desired

When you allow these biscotti to dry completely, they are great dunkers in an afternoon cup of tea. They can also be made without the stevia; they won't be sweet, but they will still be very satisfying.

  2 cups raw unsalted organic almonds

  ¼ cup unsweetened organic coconut flakes

  3 tablespoons organic cocoa powder

  2 tablespoons organic chia seeds

  1 large organic egg from a pasture-raised chicken, at room temperature

  ¼ cup organic coconut oil

  1 tablespoon granulated organic stevia

  1 teaspoon baking soda

Combine the almonds, coconut, cocoa powder, and chia seeds in the bowl of a food processor fitted with a metal blade. Pulse until the mixture resembles very fine crumbs.

Scrape the mixture into a medium mixing bowl. Add the egg, coconut oil, stevia, and baking soda, beating to combine well.

Preheat the oven to 375°F.

Scrape the dough from the bowl and, using your

hands, form it into a loaf about an inch thick. Wrap in plastic wrap and refrigerate for about 30 minutes, or until firmed slightly.

Remove the dough from the refrigerator, unwrap, and cut crosswise into 8 to 10 bars of equal size.

Lay the cookies about 1 inch apart on an ungreased cookie sheet. Place in the preheated oven and bake for about 10 minutes, or until the dough has firmed somewhat and begun to color around the edges.

You can either remove the cookies from the oven and serve them warm and soft or, for a crisper cookie, turn the oven off and let them stay in the cooling oven to dry slightly. If you prefer very crisp biscotti, when the oven has cooled, remove the cookies and transfer to a wire rack to rest for 12 hours at room temperature.

Ricotta Mousse

Serves 4
Time required: About 15 minutes

This is a light and refreshing dessert that can also be made with ½ cup of dark (at least 80% cacao) chocolate chips, alone or in combination with the berries. It travels well, so it is a terrific low-carb dessert to take to a potluck or a summer barbecue.

2 cups Ricotta Cheese (page 198)

¼ cup organic heavy cream from grass-fed cows

2 tablespoons granulated organic stevia, or more to taste

¾ cup organic blueberries or raspberries

1 teaspoon freshly grated organic orange zest

Organic cocoa powder for dusting

Combine the Ricotta Cheese, cream, and stevia in the bowl of a food processor fitted with a metal blade and process until very light and smooth.

Scrape the mixture into a medium mixing bowl. Gently stir in the berries and the orange zest. Spoon an equal portion into each of four small dessert bowls. Dust with cocoa powder and serve.

May be stored, covered and refrigerated, for a day or two.

Almond Panna Cotta

Serves 4 to 6

Time required: About 30 minutes, plus 4 hours or more for chilling

This light dessert always impresses! If you really want to fancy it up, puree a cup of blueberries, spoon an equal portion of the puree on each serving plate, then garnish with whole berries and a mint leaf.

1 cup unsweetened organic almond milk

1 cup organic heavy cream from grass-fed cows, divided

1½ teaspoons unflavored gelatin

1 tablespoon granulated organic stevia

1 teaspoon pure organic almond extract

½ cup organic blueberries

4–6 organic mint leaves

Combine the almond milk with ½ cup of the heavy cream in a small heavy-bottom saucepan over low heat. Heat for about 6 minutes, or until bubbles form around the edge of the pan.

While the almond milk is heating, pour the remaining ½ cup of heavy cream into a medium heatproof mixing bowl. Add the gelatin and let stand to soften.

When the almond milk mixture is hot, pour it over the gelatin mixture. Add the stevia and stir until completely blended.

Set aside to cool to room temperature. Then stir in the almond extract. Pour an equal portion of the mixture into either four 4-ounce ramekins or six smaller ramekins.

Cover each ramekin with plastic wrap, and transfer to the refrigerator. Let chill for at least 4 hours, or until firm.

To serve, invert each ramekin onto a dessert plate. Garnish with a few berries and a mint leaf. If the panna cotta does not easily slip out of the ramekins, wrap the ramekins in a wet hot towel for a few seconds.

Serve immediately.

DRINKS

Matcha Smoothie

Serves 2

Time required: About 5 minutes

This smoothie is a wonderful afternoon energy booster—refreshing, delectable, and so good for you. You can add a couple of ice cubes to it while blending for a bit of slushiness in the final drink.

- 2 large organic Persian cucumbers
- ¼ cup organic mint leaves
- ½ teaspoon organic matcha (green tea powder)
- 2 cups chilled organic coconut water

Chop the cucumbers and place them in a blender. Add the mint leaves, matcha, and coconut water and process until very smooth.

Pour into two glasses and serve.

Afternoon Pick-Me-Up

Serves 2
Time required: About 7 minutes

Green and smooth and slightly tart, this drink is just the right thing to wake you up in the late afternoon. If you've limited your carbs during the day, you might splurge and add half a small banana for a little more texture and sweetness. But if you do, remember to keep the remainder of your carb intake low.

1 organic avocado, peeled and seeded

2 cups chopped trimmed organic kale leaves

1 cup chilled organic coconut water

1 cup chilled organic unsweetened almond milk

2 tablespoons chopped organic mint leaves

1 tablespoon chopped organic ginger

1 teaspoon freshly squeezed organic lime juice

Combine all ingredients in a blender. Process until smooth and creamy.

Place a few ice cubes in each of two large glasses and divide the mixture between the two.

Serve immediately.

Hibiscus Tea

Serves 4

Time required: About 15 minutes

Hot or iced hibiscus tea is frequently the beverage of choice for people who are fasting. We love its fruitiness and its ability to refresh on a hot summer day. Ginger and herbs seem to be great partners for this wonderfully healing tea.

⅓ cup dried organic hibiscus flowers (see Note)

7 organic basil leaves

½-inch knob organic ginger, peeled

1 tablespoon freshly squeezed organic lime juice

Granulated organic stevia to taste (optional)

4 organic mint sprigs for garnish (optional)

Combine the hibiscus flowers, basil, ginger, and 4 cups cold water in a medium saucepan. Place over medium heat and bring to a boil. Immediately remove from the heat, cover, and set aside to steep for 15 minutes.

Stir in the lime juice and, if using, the stevia. Strain into a teapot or, if serving chilled, a pitcher. If the latter, either add ice or refrigerate for a couple of hours to chill.

Serve garnished with a mint sprig if desired.

NOTE: If they're available, you can use fresh organically grown hibiscus flowers instead of dried leaves to make the tea. Remove the green part at the base of the flower along with the pistil (the thin thread in the center that holds the pollen) and proceed just as you would with dried leaves.

Gingerade

Makes about 2 quarts
Time required: About 40 minutes

This is a very, very old recipe that was used as a pick-me-up during times of hot, hard farm work. It should not be sweet; the refreshing tang of ginger is what serves to revitalize and refresh. It is a delicious drink to serve at backyard parties and beach picnics.

- 6 ounces organic ginger, peeled and chopped
- Peel of 3 organic lemons, cut into thin strips
- Peel of 1 organic orange, cut into thin strips
- Juice of 3 organic lemons
- Juice of 1 organic orange
- Granulated organic stevia to taste
- Organic mint sprigs for garnish (optional)

Combine the ginger with the citrus peels in a large saucepan. Pour 2 quarts of boiling water over the mixture, cover, and set aside to steep for 30 minutes, or until the liquid is very fragrant.

Add the citrus juice and the stevia, stirring to blend. Add only a tiny bit of the stevia at a time and taste after each addition. The beverage should be quite gingery and tart.

When ready to serve, fill a large pitcher with ice and pour the gingerade over it. If desired, place a mint sprig in each glass as you serve.

Powerhouse Coffee

Serves 2

Time required: About 5 minutes

This coffee drink can start your day off with a bang or end it with a sizzle. It is rather like a delicious, rich cappuccino that turns into an enticing dessert. It is important to use a high-speed blender such as a Vitamix so that all the ingredients emulsify into a creamy mixture.

- 2 cups hot strong brewed organic coffee
- 3 tablespoons finely grated organic dark chocolate, at least 80% cacao
- 2 tablespoons organic unsalted butter from grass-fed cows, at room temperature
- 1 tablespoon MCT oil (see page 256)
- 2 tablespoons organic heavy cream from grass-fed cows
- Organic ground cinnamon for garnish

Combine the coffee, chocolate, butter, and oil in a high-speed blender. Process for a minute or so, or until the mixture is smooth and creamy.

Pour into two warmed coffee cups, then spoon 1 tablespoon of heavy cream into each cup and sprinkle with ground cinnamon.

Serve immediately.

Turmeric Milk Shake

Serves 2

Time required: About 7 minutes

This drink is best made with fresh turmeric and ginger in a high-speed blender such as a Vitamix. Still, you should grate the turmeric and ginger to ensure that the finished drink will be smooth and creamy. You can use almond milk and coconut oil in place of the coconut milk and avocado oil. If you have fresh coconut, it will add a lovely flavor, though it's not necessary.

3¼ cups organic unsweetened coconut milk, chilled

2 tablespoons organic avocado oil

5-inch piece fresh organic turmeric root, peeled and grated, or 2 teaspoons organic ground turmeric

1-inch piece organic ginger, peeled and grated, or 1 teaspoon organic ground ginger

¼ cup unsweetened shredded or flaked organic coconut

1 teaspoon pure organic vanilla extract

1 teaspoon freshly grated organic orange zest, plus more for garnish

½ teaspoon organic ground cinnamon

4 ice cubes

Combine the coconut milk and avocado oil in the jar of a high-speed blender. Process to just blend.

Add the turmeric, ginger, coconut, vanilla, orange zest, and cinnamon and process to just combine. Add the ice cubes and process on high until the mixture is smooth, thick, and bright yellow.

Pour an equal portion into each of two tall glasses. Sprinkle the top with orange zest and serve.

Conclusion

We Need You

Invisible threads are the strongest ties.

— Friedrich Nietzsche

The world as we have created it is a process of our thinking. It cannot be changed without changing our thinking.

— Albert Einstein

We're all searching for the same things in life. We want happiness, success, and a sense of purpose. We want to be physically and mentally fit. We want to enjoy deep interpersonal bonds. We want our lives to have direction and meaning. But through bad habits and self-sabotaging behaviors, we can often get in our own way when we attempt to achieve these goals.

When we mindlessly cave into cravings, impulses, and fears, we lose at life. We substitute anger for love and narcissism for empathy. We embrace negativity and pessimism at the expense of positivity and optimism. We close ourselves off from our families, our friends, and the world. The painful and regrettable truth: we have become lonely people in an increasingly isolating world. And we devote our time and energy to activities that we know won't bring us what we seek.

This cannot be the way forward. We need connection — to our surroundings, to others, and to our own conscious thoughts and actions. It's that simple.

TIES THAT BIND

The world's population is almost eight billion, so it's hard to imagine that feelings of isolation and loneliness still affect so many of us. We're so much more similar than we are different, despite what the media would have you believe. We have so much to gain and learn from one another. But as we know, multiple influences interfere with our ability to use our prefrontal cortices. When this happens, we resort to impulsivity and fear. We see others as inferior because of their culture, sex, or ideology. We judge and criticize. We begin to believe that we are all alone in facing an uncertain, unpredictable, and frightening world, and we become increasingly pessimistic about the future.

What if we decided to take a different approach to life by embracing the power of interpersonal relationships and all the benefits they confer? We would refuse to participate in the endless cycle of unnecessary distress, anger, insecurity, and partisanship, instead spending our time and energy strengthening our close relationships. In the bigger picture, these ties to our friends, families, and society as a whole are essential for everything we've discussed in this book. We simply can't escape disconnection syndrome on our own.

Yes, it's true that our neighbors can become strangers, our families distant, and our friendships superficial. But this reality is anything but necessary. Humans are engineered for connection; our brains crave it. Our hearts ache for it. We thrive when we're linked. In his bestseller *The Hidden Life of Trees,* Peter Wohlleben writes, "If you 'help' individual trees by getting rid of their supposed competition, the remaining trees are bereft." Humans are no different. Cooperation has been key to our survival as a species. We are happier and longer-lived when we're connected. Our relationships to others give us a strong root system and provide the stability we need to flourish. We cannot prosper from this incredible wellspring of power if we only look at others as rivals.

LESSONS FROM THE LONGEST STUDY ON HAPPINESS

It's easy to see the need for interpersonal connection when we approach the subject from an evolutionary perspective. Hunter-gatherers relied on one another to share knowledge and protection. But modern technology reduces our need to rely on others. Our environment is engineered to promote and provide self-sufficiency. However, our connections to other people turn out to have many important benefits besides keeping us informed and safe.

For more than eighty years, researchers in the Harvard Study of Adult Development have been studying the secrets to a good long life, finding the power of community to be among the most critical factors.[1] They first started recording data back in 1938, during the Great Depression, following the health of 268 Harvard undergraduate males. The study is currently led by Dr. Robert Waldinger, a psychiatrist at Massachusetts General Hospital and a professor of psychiatry at Harvard Medical School. His TEDx talk on the subject—"What Makes a Good Life?"—has been viewed more than twenty-eight million times. Dr. Waldinger and his team have been at the helm of multiple significant research publications over the years that show us how much we gain from the presence of others in our lives.

One study conducted by this group specifically looked at whether the strength of interpersonal bonds was linked to health outcomes.[2] The researchers examined eighty-one couples, asking them questions about their well-being and testing their memory. They also measured attachment, which is a psychological term defined as a "deep and enduring emotional bond that connects one person to another across time and space."[3] After two and a half years, the researchers reevaluated the couples on their memory and well-being. The couples with strong attachment had less depression, better mood, and greater overall life satisfaction than those with weak attachment. What's more, the women in this group had better memory.

If our mental health is improved when we have strong bonds with others, is it worsened when our relationships are poor? The same Harvard researchers investigated this question by reviewing whether the quality of relationships between child siblings correlated with the development of depression as adults.[4] The study demonstrated that poor sibling relationships before the age of twenty were highly correlated with an increased risk of major depression and the use of mood-altering drugs later in life. Strong, enriching relationships are sustenance, like food and water. And best of all, it doesn't take much to improve our bonds with those we care about. Sometimes it's as simple as picking up the phone.

AUSTIN'S LESSON IN THE ICU

During my medical residency, when I was working in the intensive care unit (ICU), all my patients were critically ill. The mood could easily have become bleak. But these were also some of the most meaningful times in my medical training. In the ICU, I had the honor of providing care for patients as they approached their final hours. And as different as all their lives had been before they came to the hospital, once they were there, they shared a similar desire. They wanted to be with their closest friends and family at the end—that was what mattered most. Confronted with some of the most emotional reunions I've ever witnessed, I stopped thinking about what to eat for my next meal, where to go on my next day off, and even what to do for the rest of my life. Instead, I called my parents and my sister, took the time to see an old friend, and paused to think about all the people I care about. There are so many reasons to cling to a narrative of isolation, but in the end, that's not the story I want to live. My patients gave me many gifts—but I'll always consider myself especially lucky for the gift of this understanding.

Social relationships aren't just a way to produce happiness. As you know by now, these bonds are strongly linked with the length of our life spans and our risk of illness. The Harvard study is one of many taking place today that reveal the power of personal connection over our health. A study conducted in Japan, for example, found that Japanese elders who partook in social activities had a 32 percent lower risk of dying over a three-year period than those who were less socially engaged.[5] What's more (and somewhat contrary to what you might think), those with strong social ties appeared to be four times *less* likely to contract the common cold.[6] Social integration has also been shown to protect against coronary artery disease; those without social integration may suffer an almost fourfold increased risk of developing it as well as a higher chance of dying from it. The authors were so stunned by their results that they concluded that the negative health impact of low social integration "was of similar magnitude as that of smoking."[7]

Much is written these days about the incredible health and longevity of people living in the so-called Blue Zones.[8] But what's not commonly known is that they may owe a good portion of their robustness not to the food they eat or the exercise they get but to their social connectedness. Their interpersonal bonds. Simple as that. And no, they are not making them on the internet.

WHO IS WRITING YOUR STORY?

We all live on the same blue sphere. And while the opportunities, challenges, and events in our lives may vary, we share the same major plot points. We're born, we live, then we die. The genre of the story can be tragedy, comedy, or even action thriller. Much of this has little to do with our experiences and a lot to do with how we interpret them. We don't have to be passive characters in our stories. We can become the authors of our own scripts. They should not be written by those who profit from keeping us unwell and unsatisfied. **Either you control your brain or others will do it for you.**

Yes, we will each face momentous trials and tribulations during which we must fight against the despair and anger within our heads. But most of the battles for our minds are being played out in the spaces between these major life events. It's the little things—the food we choose to eat, the technology we use, the news we subscribe to, the media we consume, the relationships we choose to foster—that will determine whether our brains belong to us or to those who seek to hijack them. This is a wake-up call. It is a chance to see the world for what it is and ask whether your story is your own. If you find it is not, this is your chance to take it back.

You have to make a decision. Will you let others determine your fate, allowing them to rewire your brain? Or will you instead harness the power of neuroplasticity for your own gain and rebuild your brain for the life you want? We believe that disconnection syndrome can be healed on an individual and a societal level. But we can't do this alone. We need one another. *We need you.*

Acknowledgments

This book has been a lot more than a labor of love. When we came together as father and son, we grew together as coauthors and partners in scripting an important message that transcended our relationship. Our experience unfolded in ways we never could have imagined at the start of this project. And we are much more connected than ever before. We thank each other for pulling through what was a challenging experience—crafting a manuscript written from the perspective of two different generations, two points of view, yet one collective goal. We did it, and the journey was rewarding beyond measure.

We were not alone in this process: anyone who has ever written a book knows that it takes a force of creative, bright, and tireless people to make it happen. We owe a heartfelt thank-you to more people than we can possibly name here, because an untold number of individuals have contributed to our ways of thinking. We are indebted to all the scientists, mentors, and colleagues who have taught us so much and helped us understand the mysteries of the human brain and body. We also owe much gratitude to the patients we've cared for, who have enlightened us with their stories and showed us how to be better doctors. You provide insights that cannot be found elsewhere. This book is as much yours as it is ours. And now we would like to thank a few selected people who contributed directly to this manuscript.

Kristin Loberg, our collaborator, accepted the challenge of creating a work written by two authors. Thank you for being the team player that you are and making this a magical experience. Our literary agent, Bonnie Solow, has played a central role in the manifestation of this project. Thank you, Bonnie, not just for your agency accomplishments but also for your gracious guidance and support in so many other areas. You always go beyond the call of duty.

We are deeply grateful to Proton Enterprises, under the leadership of James Murphy, for skillfully overseeing the multiple moving parts of our messaging process. Heartfelt appreciation goes especially to Andrew Luer, not only for your ability to develop and execute novel ideas but also for your oversight of the wide scope of our outreach platform.

Thanks go to our friends at Digital Natives for their continued skill and dedication in handling our digital media efforts.

Leize Perlmutter, wife and mother, thank you for always being available to lovingly share suggestions that have proved so helpful in the formulation of this work.

Thanks to the indefatigable team at Little, Brown Spark that has championed this book. A special thanks goes to Tracy Behar, our gifted editor, with her exceptional skill for keeping us on message, knowing where to cut or clarify, and ensuring that the manuscript is accessible and cogent. Your editorial mastery made this a much better book through all its iterations. Thanks also to Michael Pietsch, Reagan Arthur, Ian Straus, Jessica Chun, Juliana Horbachevsky, Craig Young, Pamela Brown, Sabrina Callahan, Barbara Clark, and Julianna Lee. It's been a pleasure to work with such a dedicated, professional group.

Thanks to Judith Choate, who created the original and tasty recipes in her own kitchen. They not only abide by our rules but also make cooking fun.

And finally, Austin would like to make the following acknowledgment: I so appreciate James Murphy, John D'Orazio, and Mitch Leonardi for your curiosity, support, insight, and encouragement as we navigate life's most challenging questions together. I'm also grateful to Rachel Costantino for reminding me to enjoy the wonder of the world around me. Thank you for your encouragement and for providing balance in my life.

Illustration Credits

Page 48: John M. Harlow, "Recovery from the Passage of an Iron Bar through the Head," *Publications of the Massachusetts Medical Society* 2, no. 3 (1868): 327–47. Reprinted by David Clapp & Son (1869).

Page 70: Kalev H. Leetaru, "Culturomics 2.0: Forecasting Large-Scale Human Behavior Using Global News Media Tone in Time and Space," *First Monday* 16, no. 9 (September 5, 2011). Available at: https://firstmonday .org/ojs/index.php/fm/article/view/3663/3040>. Accessed May 23, 2019. Reprinted with permission from Dr. Leetaru.

Page 106: Adapted from Claire Pearson and Zaheer Hussain, "Smartphone Use, Addiction, Narcissism, and Personality: A Mixed Methods Investigation," *International Journal of Cyber Behavior, Psychology and Learning* 5, no. 1 (January–March 2015): 17–32.

Page 192: Adapted from Seung-Schik Yoo et al., "The Human Emotional Brain without Sleep—a Prefrontal Amygdala Disconnect," *Current Biology* 17, no. 20 (October 23, 2007): R877–78.

Page 210: © Randy Glasbergen. Glasbergen.com. Reprinted with permission.

Notes

The following is a list of scientific papers and other references that you might find helpful if you want to learn more about some of the ideas and concepts expressed in this book. These materials can also open doors for further research and inquiry. For access to more studies and an ongoing updated list of references, please visit BrainWashBook.com.

Introduction

1. Pew Research Center, "Political Polarization in the American Public: How Increasing Ideological Uniformity and Partisan Antipathy Affect Politics, Compromise and Everyday Life," June 12, 2014, http://assets .pewresearch.org/wp-content/uploads/sites/5/2014/06/6-12-2014 -Political-Polarization-Release.pdf.
2. For data about chronic disease in America, see the Centers for Disease Control and Prevention's National Center for Chronic Disease Prevention and Health Promotion website at https://www.cdc.gov/chronicdisease /resources/infographic/chronic-diseases.htm (accessed May 16, 2019).
3. National Association of Chronic Disease Directors, "Why We Need Public Health to Improve Healthcare," https://www.chronicdisease.org /page/whyweneedph2imphc (accessed August 4, 2019); see also Centers for Disease Control and Prevention, "Health and Economic Costs of

Chronic Diseases," https://www.cdc.gov/chronicdisease/about/costs/index .htm (accessed July 19, 2019).

4. World Health Organization, "Noncommunicable Diseases and Their Risk Factors," https://www.who.int/ncds/en/ (accessed May 16, 2019).

Chapter 1

1. "Ericsson Mobility Report: 70 Percent of World's Population Using Smartphones by 2020," press release, June 3, 2015, https://www.ericsson .com/en/press-releases/2015/6/ericsson-mobility-report-70-percent -of-worlds-population-using-smartphones-by-2020.

2. For data on digital media use, see Nielsen.com.

3. "Americans Spend Nearly Half of Their Waking Hours (42 percent) Looking at a Screen, It's Been Revealed by New Research," press release, August 13, 2018, survey conducted by OnePoll on behalf of CooperVi- sion, https://coopervision.com/our-company/news-center/press-release/ americans-spend-nearly-half-their-waking-hours-42-percent.

4. S. C. Curtin et al., "Recent Increases in Injury Mortality Among Chil- dren and Adolescents Aged 10–19 Years in the United States: 1999– 2016," *Natl. Vital Stat. Rep.* 67, no. 4 (June 2018): 1–16.

5. National Center for Health Statistics, *Health, United States, 2010: With Special Feature on Death and Dying*, table 95 (Hyattsville, MD: US Department of Health and Human Services, 2011): 319–21.

6. M. Markota et al., "Benzodiazepine Use in Older Adults: Dangers, Management, and Alternative Therapies," *Mayo Clin. Proc.* 91, no. 11 (November 2016): 1632–39.

7. See the National Sleep Foundation at SleepFoundation.org.

8. V. Poznyak and D. Rekve, eds., *Global Status Report on Alcohol and Health 2018* (Geneva: World Health Organization, 2018).

9. Poznyak and Rekve, *Global Status Report*.

10. "New Cigna Study Reveals Loneliness at Epidemic Levels in America," press release, May 1, 2018, https://cigna.newshq.businesswire.com/press -release/new-cigna-study-reveals-loneliness-epidemic-levels-america ?WT.z_nav=newsroom%2Fnews-releases%2F2018%2Fnew-cigna -study-reveals-loneliness-at-epidemic-levels-in-america%3BBody %3Bhttp%3A%2F%2Fcigna.newshq.businesswire.com%2Fpress

-release%2Fnew-cigna-study-reveals-loneliness-epidemic-levels
-america.

11. "New Cigna Study."

12. R. Micha et al., "Association Between Dietary Factors and Mortality from Heart Disease, Stroke, and Type 2 Diabetes in the United States," *JAMA* 317, no. 9 (March 7, 2017): 912–24.

13. H. Waters and M. Graf, *America's Obesity Crisis: The Health and Economic Costs of Excess Weight* (Santa Monica, CA: Milken Institute, October 26, 2018), https://www.milkeninstitute.org/reports/americas -obesity-crisis-health-and-economic-costs-excess-weight.

Chapter 2

1. Sharon Begley, *Train Your Mind, Change Your Brain: How a New Science Reveals Our Extraordinary Potential to Transform Ourselves* (New York: Ballantine, 2007).

2. G. Weinstein et al., "Serum Brain-Derived Neurotrophic Factor and the Risk for Dementia: The Framingham Heart Study," *JAMA Neurol.* 71, no. 1 (January 2014): 55–61.

3. See the interview with Dr. Bredesen at DrPerlmutter.com.

4. The famous "triune brain theory" was originally developed by American neuroscientist Dr. Paul MacLean in the 1960s. See J. D. Newman and J. C. Harris's review of his works: "The Scientific Contributions of Paul D. MacLean (1913–2007)," *J. Nerv. Ment. Dis.* 197, no. 1 (January 2009): 3–5.

5. J. S. Feinstein et al., "The Human Amygdala and the Induction and Experience of Fear," *Curr. Biol.* 21, no. 1 (January 2011): 34–38.

6. J. B. MacKinnon, "The Strange Brain of the World's Greatest Solo Climber," *Nautilus* 039, August 11, 2016.

7. M. J. Kim et al., "The Structural and Functional Connectivity of the Amygdala: From Normal Emotion to Pathological Anxiety," *Behavioral Brain Research* 223, no. 2 (October 2011): 403–10.

8. J. A. Rosenkranz, E. R. Venheim, and M. Padival, "Chronic Stress Causes Amygdala Hyperexcitability in Rodents," *Biol. Psychiatry* 67, no. 12 (June 2010): 1128–36.

9. For a summary of Phineas Gage's life and lessons, see the *Smithsonian*

article about him by Steve Twomey: "Phineas Gage: Neuroscience's Most Famous Patient" (January 2010), https://www.smithsonianmag .com/history/phineas-gage-neurosciences-most-famous-patient -11390067/.

10. The observations noted by Dr. Williams landed in published statements by one Dr. John Harlow, who took over Gage's case. See J. M. Harlow, "Passage of an Iron Rod through the Head," *Boston Med. Surg. J.* 39, no. 20 (December 13, 1848): 389–93.

11. Harlow, "Passage of an Iron Rod"; also see J. M. Harlow, "Recovery from the Passage of an Iron Bar through the Head," *Publ. Mass. Med. Soc.* 2 (1868): 327–47.

12. M. Ironside et al., "Effect of Prefrontal Cortex Stimulation on Regulation of Amygdala Response to Threat in Individuals with Trait Anxiety: A Randomized Clinical Trial," *JAMA Psychiatry* (October 2018), doi: 10.1001/jamapsychiatry.2018.2172 [Epub ahead of print].

13. N. J. Kelley et al., "Stimulating Self-Regulation: A Review of Non-Invasive Brain Stimulation Studies of Goal-Directed Behavior," *Front. Behav. Neurosci.* 12 (January 2019): 337.

14. A. T. Park et al., "Amygdala–Medial Prefrontal Cortex Connectivity Relates to Stress and Mental Health in Early Childhood," *Soc. Cogn. Affect. Neurosci.* 13, no. 4 (April 2018): 430–39.

15. Park et al., "Amygdala–Medial Prefrontal Cortex Connectivity."

Chapter 3

1. A. F. T. Arnsten, "Stress Signalling Pathways that Impair Prefrontal Cortex Structure and Function," *Nat. Rev. Neurosci.* 10, no. 6 (June 2009): 410–22.

2. Arnsten, "Stress Signalling Pathways."

3. A. F. T. Arnsten, "Stress Weakens Prefrontal Networks: Molecular Insults to Higher Cognition," *Nat. Neurosci.* 18, no. 10 (October 2015): 1376–85.

4. A. Nagano-Saito et al., "Stress-Induced Dopamine Release in Human Medial Prefrontal Cortex — 18F-fallypride/PET Study in Healthy Volunteers," *Synapse* 67, no. 12 (December 2013): 821–30.

5. International Data Corporation, "Always Connected: How Smart-

phones and Social Keep Us Engaged," https://www.nu.nl/files/IDC
-Facebook%20Always%20Connected%20%281%29.pdf (accessed May
19, 2019).

6. International Data Corporation, "Always Connected."

7. "Kellogg Reveals Results of Monumental Breakfast Survey," press release,
June 22, 2011, http://newsroom.kelloggcompany.com/news-releases
?item=76379.

8. J. E. Gangwisch et al., "High Glycemic Index Diet as a Risk Factor for
Depression: Analyses from the Women's Health Initiative," *Am. J. Clin.
Nutr.* 102, no. 2 (August 2015): 454–63.

9. N. D. Mehta et al., "Inflammation Negatively Correlates with
Amygdala-Ventromedial Prefrontal Functional Connectivity in Asso-
ciation with Anxiety in Patients with Depression: Preliminary Results,"
Brain Behav. Immun. 73 (October 2018): 725–30.

10. T. K. Inagaki et al., "Inflammation Selectively Enhances Amygdala
Activity to Socially Threatening Images," *Neuroimage* 59, no. 4 (February 2012): 3222–26.

11. E. Stice, K. S. Burger, and S. Yokum, "Relative Ability of Fat and Sugar
Tastes to Activate Reward, Gustatory, and Somatosensory Regions,"
Am. J. Clin. Nutr. 98, no. 6 (December 2013): 1377–84.

12. N. D. Volkow, R. A. Wise, and R. Baler, "The Dopamine Motive System: Implications for Drug and Food Addiction," *Nat. Rev. Neurosci.*
18, no. 12 (November 2017): 741–52.

13. American Psychological Association, "Stress in America: The State of
Our Nation" (November 1, 2017), https://www.apa.org/news/press
/releases/stress/2017/state-nation.pdf.

14. A. Mitchell et al., "The Modern News Consumer: News Attitudes and
Practices in the Digital Era," Pew Research Center, July 7, 2016, https://
www.journalism.org/2016/07/07/the-modern-news-consumer/.

15. Mitchell et al., "The Modern News Consumer."

16. Mitchell et al., "The Modern News Consumer."

17. American Psychological Association, "Stress in America."

18. J. Poushter, "Worldwide, People Divided on Whether Life Today Is
Better Than in the Past," Pew Research Center, December 5, 2017,
https://www.pewresearch.org/global/2017/12/05/worldwide-people
-divided-on-whether-life-today-is-better-than-in-the-past/.

19. J. Gramlich, "5 Facts about Crime in the U.S.," Pew Research Center, January 3, 2019, https://www.pewresearch.org/fact-tank/2019/01/03/5 -facts-about-crime-in-the-u-s/.

20. M. Roser and M. Nagdy, "Optimism and Pessimism," OurWorldInData .org, https://ourworldindata.org/optimism-pessimism (accessed May 19, 2019).

21. "The Burden of Stress in America," survey conducted by the NPR/Robert Wood Johnson Foundation/Harvard School of Public Health, 2014, https://media.npr.org/documents/2014/july/npr_rwfj_harvard_stress _poll.pdf.

22. A. Szabo, "Negative Psychological Effects of Watching the News in the Television: Relaxation or Another Intervention May Be Needed to Buffer Them!" *Int. J. Behav. Med.* 14, no. 2 (2007): 57–62.

23. K. Leetaru, "Culturomics 2.0: Forecasting Large-Scale Human Behavior Using Global News Media Tone in Time and Space," *First Monday* 16, no. 9 (September 5, 2011).

24. S. Vosoughi, D. Roy, and S. Aral, "The Spread of True and False News Online," MIT Initiative on the Digital Economy Research Brief, 2017, http://ide.mit.edu/sites/default/files/publications/2017%20IDE%20 Research%20Brief%20False%20News.pdf.

25. "Dig Deeper: Critical Thinking in the Digital Age," MindEdge, 2018, https://www2.mindedge.com/page/dig-deeper.

26. "Labor Day Survey: 51% of U.S. Employees Overall Satisfied with Their Job," press release, August 29, 2018, https://www.conference -board.org/press/pressdetail.cfm?pressid=7528.

27. C. Kong, "Bored at Work," Robert Half blog, October 19, 2017, https:// www.roberthalf.com/blog/management-tips/bored-at-work.

28. "State of the Global Workplace," Gallup, 2017, https://www.gallup .com/workplace/238079/state-global-workplace-2017.aspx?utm_source= 2013StateofGlobalWorkplaceReport&utm_medium=2013SOGWRepo rtLandingPage&utm_campaign=2013StateofGlobalReport_Redirectto 2017page&utm_content=download2017now_textlink.

29. "Mind the Workplace," report by Mental Health America, 2017, https:// www.mentalhealthamerica.net/sites/default/files/Mind%20the%20 Workplace%20-%20MHA%20Workplace%20Health%20Survey%20 2017%20FINAL.pdf.

30. "Nielsen Total Audience Report: Q1 2018," https://www.nielsen.com/us/en/insights/report/2018/q1-2018-total-audience-report/.

Chapter 4

1. T. Harris, "How Technology Is Hijacking Your Mind—from a Magician and Google Design Ethicist," *Thrive Global,* May 18, 2016.
2. C. Cheng and A. Y. Li, "Internet Addiction Prevalence and Quality of (Real) Life: A Meta-Analysis of 31 Nations Across Seven World Regions," *Cyberpsychol. Behav. Soc. Netw.* 17, no. 12 (December 2014): 755–60.
3. Nathan McDonald, "Digital in 2018: World's Internet Users Pass the 4 Billion Mark," We Are Social, January 30, 2018, https://wearesocial.com/us/blog/2018/01/global-digital-report-2018.
4. J. T. F. Lau et al., "Incidence and Predictive Factors of Internet Addiction Among Chinese Secondary School Students in Hong Kong: A Longitudinal Study," *Soc. Psychiatry Psychiatr. Epidemiol.* 52, no. 6 (June 2017): 657–67.
5. M. A. Moreno et al., "Problematic Internet Use Among US Youth: A Systematic Review," *Arch. Pediatr. Adolesc. Med.* 165, no. 9 (September 2011): 797–805.
6. Y. Zhou et al., "Gray Matter Abnormalities in Internet Addiction: A Voxel-Based Morphometry Study," *Eur. J. Radiol.* 79, no. 1 (July 2011): 92–95. See also R. Z. Goldstein and N. D. Volkow, "Dysfunction of the Prefrontal Cortex in Addiction: Neuroimaging Findings and Clinical Implications," *Nat. Rev. Neurosci.* 12, no. 11 (October 2011): 652–69.
7. Y. Zhou et al., "Altered Default Network Resting-State Functional Connectivity in Adolescents with Internet Gaming Addiction," *PLoS One* 8, no. 3 (March 26, 2013): e59902.
8. R. J. Dwyer, K. Kushlev, and E. W. Dunn, "Smartphone Use Undermines Enjoyment of Face-to-Face Social Interactions," *J. Exp. Soc. Psychol.* 78 (September 2018): 233–39.
9. Shalini Misra, Lulu Cheng, Jamie Genevie, and Miao Yuan, "The iPhone Effect: The Quality of In-Person Social Interactions in the Presence of Mobile Devices," *Environment and Behavior* 48, no. 2 (2016).

10. J. Schroeder et al., "Handshaking Promotes Cooperative Dealmaking," Harvard Business School NOM Unit Working Paper 14-117, May 2014, available at SSRN (Social Science Research Network): https://ssrn.com/abstract=2443674 or http://dx.doi.org/10.2139/ssrn.2443674.

11. S. T. Asma, "This Friendship Has Been Digitized," op-ed, *New York Times,* March 23, 2019, https://www.nytimes.com/2019/03/23/opinion/this-friendship-has-been-digitized.html.

12. For more about Dr. Lisa Strohman, see her website at DrLisaStrohman.com.

13. J. D. Elhai et al., "Problematic Smartphone Use: A Conceptual Overview and Systematic Review of Relations with Anxiety and Depression Psychopathology," *J. Affect. Disord.* 207 (January 2017): 251–59.

14. Y. S. Cheng et al., "Internet Addiction and Its Relationship with Suicidal Behaviors: A Meta-Analysis of Multinational Observational Studies," *J. Clin. Psychiatry* 79, no. 4 (June 2018): 17r11761.

15. D. L. Clark, J. L. Raphael, and A. L. McGuire, "HEADS: Social Media Screening in Adolescent Primary Care," *Pediatrics* 141, no. 6 (June 2018).

16. ABC News Australia, "Internet-Addicted South Korean Children Sent to Digital Detox Boot Camp," viewable at https://youtu.be/YuT_RAugJu0.

17. Matt Cutts's Twitter account: @MattCutts.

18. For all the statistics about social media trends and use, download *Social: GlobalWebIndex's Flagship Report on the Latest Trends in Social Media* (2018) at https://www.globalwebindex.com/hubfs/Downloads/Social-H2-2018-report.pdf.

19. Saima Salin, "How Much Time Do You Spend on Social Media? Research Says 142 Minutes per Day," *Digital Information World,* January 4, 2019 (www.digitalinformationworld.com).

20. *Social: GlobalWebIndex's Flagship Report.*

21. Chamath Palihapitiya's interview was posted by Tim Hains on December 11, 2017, under the title "Former Facebook Exec: Social Media Is Ripping Our Social Fabric Apart," at https://www.realclearpolitics.com/video/2017/12/11/fmr_facebook_exec_social_media_is_ripping_our_social_fabric_apart.html.

22. J. R. Corrigan et al., "How Much Is Social Media Worth? Estimating the Value of Facebook by Paying Users to Stop Using It," *PLoS One* 13, no. 12 (December 2018): e0207101.

23. Happiness Research Institute, "The Facebook Experiment," 2015, at www.happinessresearchinstitute.com/publications.

24. M. G. Hunt et al., "No More FOMO: Limiting Social Media Decreases Loneliness and Depression," *J. Soc. Clin. Psychol.* 37, no. 10 (November 2018): 751–68.

25. B. A. Primack et al., "Social Media Use and Perceived Social Isolation Among Young Adults in the U.S.," *Am. J. Prev. Med.* 53, no. 1 (July 2017): 1–8.

26. P. Verduyn et al., "Passive Facebook Usage Undermines Affective Well-Being: Experimental and Longitudinal Evidence," *J. Exp. Psychol. Gen.* 144, no. 2 (April 2015): 480–88.

27. Q. He, O. Turel, and A. Bechara, "Association of Excessive Social Media Use with Abnormal White Matter Integrity of the Corpus Callosum," *Psychiatry Res. Neuroimaging* 278 (August 2018): 42–47.

28. L. E. Sherman et al., "The Power of the Like in Adolescence: Effects of Peer Influence on Neural and Behavioral Responses to Social Media," *Psychol. Sci.* 27, no. 7 (July 2016): 1027–35.

29. Lauren E. Sherman, Leanna M. Hernandez, Patricia M. Greenfield, and Mirella Dapretto, "What the Brain 'Likes': Neural Correlates of Providing Feedback on Social Media," *Social Cognitive and Affective Neuroscience* 13, no. 7 (September 2018): 699–707.

Chapter 5

1. J. Decety and P. L. Jackson, "The Functional Architecture of Human Empathy," *Behav. Cogn. Neurosci. Rev.* 3, no. 2 (June 2004): 71–100.

2. William Ickes, *Everyday Mind Reading: Understanding What Other People Think and Feel* (Amherst, NY: Prometheus Books, 2003).

3. S. H. Konrath, E. H. O'Brien, and C. Hsing, "Changes in Dispositional Empathy in American College Students Over Time: A Meta-Analysis," *Pers. Soc. Psychol. Rev.* 15, no. 2 (May 2011): 180–98.

4. For a great review of the science of empathy in general, see H. Riess, "The Science of Empathy," *J. Patient Exp.* 4, no. 2 (June 2017): 74–77, and K. Jankowiak-Siuda and W. Zajkowski, "A Neural Model of Mechanisms of Empathy Deficits in Narcissism," *Med. Sci. Monit.* 19 (2013): 934–41.

5. D. E. Reidy et al., "Effects of Narcissistic Entitlement and Exploitativeness on Human Physical Aggression," *Pers. Individ. Dif.* 44, no. 4 (March 2008): 865–75.

6. V. Blinkhorn, M. Lyons, and L. Almond, "Drop the Bad Attitude! Narcissism Predicts Acceptance of Violent Behaviour," *Pers. Individ. Dif.* 98 (August 2016): 157–61.

7. See Dr. Campbell's site for an extensive list of his research and books on narcissism: WKeithCampbell.com.

8. David G. Taylor, "(Don't You) Wish You Were Here? Narcissism, Envy, and Sharing of Travel Photos Through Social Media: An Extended Abstract," in *Marketing at the Confluence Between Entertainment and Analytics: Proceedings of the 2016 Academy of Marketing Science (AMS) World Marketing Congress,* ed. Patricia Rossi, 821–24.

9. P. Reed et al., "Visual Social Media Use Moderates the Relationship Between Initial Problematic Internet Use and Later Narcissism," *Open Psychol. J.* 11, no. 1 (September 2018): 163–70.

10. S. J. Woodruff, S. Santarossa, and J. Lacasse, "Posting #selfie on Instagram: What Are People Talking About?" *Journal of Social Media in Society* 7, no. 1 (2018): 4–14.

11. Julia Glum, "Millennials Selfies: Young Adults Will Take More Than 25,000 Pictures of Themselves During Their Lifetimes: Report," *International Business Times,* September 22, 2015. The survey was conducted by Luster Premium White, a Boston-based company that makes teeth-whitening products.

12. R. Lull and T. M. Dickinson, "Does Television Cultivate Narcissism? Relationships Between Television Exposure, Preferences for Specific Genres, and Subclinical Narcissism," *Psychol. Pop. Media Cult.* 7, no. 1 (2018): 47–60.

13. J. N. Beadle, S. Paradiso, and D. Tranel, "Ventromedial Prefrontal Cortex Is Critical for Helping Others Who Are Suffering," *Front. Neurol.* 9 (May 2018): 288.

14. Y. Mao et al., "Reduced Frontal Cortex Thickness and Cortical Volume Associated with Pathological Narcissism," *Neuroscience* 328 (July 2016): 50–57.

15. J. T. Cheng, J. L. Tracy, and G. E. Miller, "Are Narcissists Hardy or Vulnerable? The Role of Narcissism in the Production of Stress-Related

Biomarkers in Response to Emotional Distress," *Emotion* 13, no. 6 (December 2013): 1004–11.

16. R. S. Edelstein, I. S. Yim, and J. A. Quas, "Narcissism Predicts Heightened Cortisol Reactivity to a Psychosocial Stressor in Men," *J. Res. Pers.* 44, no. 5 (October 2010): 565–72; see also David A. Reinhard et al., "Expensive Egos: Narcissistic Males Have Higher Cortisol," *PLoS One* 7, no. 1 (2012): e30858.

17. R. Rogoza, "Narcissist Unmasked. Looking for the Narcissistic Decision-Making Mechanism: A Contribution from the Big Five," *Social Psychological Bulletin* 13, no. 2 (2018).

18. P. L. Lockwood et al., "Neurocomputational Mechanisms of Prosocial Learning and Links to Empathy," *Proc. Natl. Acad. Sci. USA* 113, no. 35 (August 2016): 9763-68.

19. J. Majdanzic et al., "The Selfless Mind: How Prefrontal Involvement in Mentalizing with Similar and Dissimilar Others Shapes Empathy and Prosocial Behavior," *Cognition* 157 (December 2016): 24–38.

20. S. K. Nelson-Coffey et al., "Kindness in the Blood: A Randomized Controlled Trial of the Gene Regulatory Impact of Prosocial Behavior," *Psychoneuroendocrinology* 81 (July 2017): 8–13.

21. Using neuroimaging, Christina Karns, PhD, conducts a lot of research at the University of Oregon on the way positive emotions such as gratitude interact with altruism and generosity. Check out her website and publications at https://bdl.uoregon.edu/research/people/staff/christina -karns/.

22. See RobertWaldinger.com.

23. H. Ohira et al., "Pro-Inflammatory Cytokine Predicts Reduced Rejection of Unfair Financial Offers," *Neuro. Endocrinol. Lett.* 34, no. 1 (2013): 47–51.

24. M. Wilkes, E. Milgrom, and J. R. Hoffman, "Towards More Empathic Medical Students: A Medical Student Hospitalization Experience," *Med. Educ.* 36, no. 6 (June 2002): 528–33.

25. S. A. Batt-Rawden et al., "Teaching Empathy to Medical Students: An Updated, Systematic Review," *Acad. Med.* 88, no. 8 (August 2013): 1171–77.

Chapter 6

1. E. M. Forster, "The Machine Stops," *Oxford and Cambridge Review* (November 1909).
2. Oliver Sacks, "The Machine Stops," *The New Yorker* (February 4, 2019).
3. Numerous papers have covered the relationship between exposure to nature and human health. For a recent basic review, see M. A. Repke et al., "How Does Nature Exposure Make People Healthier?: Evidence for the Role of Impulsivity and Expanded Space Perception," *PLoS One* 13, no. 8 (August 2018): e0202246.
4. United Nations, "World's Population Increasingly Urban with More Than Half Living in Urban Areas," July 10, 2014, http://www.un.org /en/development/desa/news/population/world-urbanization-prospects -2014.html.
5. Wayne C. Zipperer and Steward T. A. Pickett, "Urban Ecology: Patterns of Population Growth and Ecological Effects," in *Encyclopedia of Life Sciences* (Chichester, UK: John Wiley & Sons, 2012), 1–8.
6. See WellLivingLab.com.
7. L. T. Stiemsma et al., "The Hygiene Hypothesis: Current Perspectives and Future Therapies," *Immunotargets Ther.* 4 (July 2015): 143–57.
8. A. Mihyang et al., "Why We Need More Nature at Work: Effects of Natural Elements and Sunlight on Employee Mental Health and Work Attitudes," *PLoS One* 11, no. 5 (May 2016): e0155614.
9. N. E. Klepeis et al., "The National Human Activity Pattern Survey (NHAPS): A Resource for Assessing Exposure to Environmental Pollutants," *J. Expo. Sci. Environ. Epidemiol.* 11 (2001): 231–52.
10. Sean Simpson, "Nine in Ten (87%) Canadians Say They're Happier When They Spend Time in Nature," Ipsos, https://www.ipsos.com/en -ca/news-polls/Canadians-happier-in-nature.
11. See RichardLouv.com.
12. O. R. McCarthy, "The Key to the Sanatoria," *J. R. Soc. Med.* 94, no. 8 (August 2001): 413–17.
13. Stephen R. Kellert and Edward O. Wilson, eds., *The Biophilia Hypothesis* (Washington, D.C.: Island Press, 1993); see also Edward O. Wilson, *Biophilia* (Boston: Harvard University Press, 1984).

14. R. S. Ulrich, "View Through a Window May Influence Recovery from Surgery," *Science* 224, no. 4647 (April 1984): 420–21.

15. R. Kjaersti, G. G. Patil, and T. Hartig, "Health Benefits of a View of Nature Through the Window: A Quasi-Experimental Study of Patients in a Residential Rehabilitation Center," *Clin. Rehabil.* 26, no. 1 (January 2012): 21–32.

16. S. Park and R. H. Mattson, "Effects of Flowering and Foliage Plants in Hospital Rooms on Patients Recovering from Abdominal Surgery," *Horttechnology* 18, no. 4 (2008): 563–68.

17. C. J. Beukeboom, D. Langeveld, and K. Tanja-Dijkstra, "Stress-Reducing Effects of Real and Artificial Nature in a Hospital Waiting Room," *J. Altern. Complement. Med.* 18, no. 4 (April 2012): 329–33.

18. B. A. Bauer et al., "Effect of the Combination of Music and Nature Sounds on Pain and Anxiety in Cardiac Surgical Patients: A Randomized Study," *Altern. Ther. Health Med.* 17, no. 4 (July–August 2011): 16–23.

19. See Shinrin-Yoku.org.

20. K. Sowndhararajan and S. Kim, "Influence of Fragrances on Human Psychophysiological Activity: With Special Reference to Human Electroencephalographic Response," *Sci. Pharm.* 84, no. 4 (November 2016): 724–52.

21. Q. Li et al., "A Forest Bathing Trip Increases Human Natural Killer Activity and Expression of Anti-Cancer Proteins in Female Subjects," *J. Biol. Regul. Homeost. Agents* 22, no. 1 (January–March 2008): 45–55.

22. Q. Li et al., "A Day Trip to a Forest Park Increases Human Natural Killer Activity and the Expression of Anti-Cancer Proteins in Male Subjects," *J. Biol. Regul. Homeost. Agents* 24, no. 2 (April–June 2010): 157–65.

23. S. Dayawansa et al., "Autonomic Responses During Inhalation of Natural Fragrance of Cedrol in Humans," *Auton. Neurosci.* 108, nos. 1–2 (October 2003): 79–86.

24. Harumi Ikei, Chorong Song, and Yoshifumi Miyazaki, "Physiological Effect of Olfactory Stimulation by Hinoki Cypress (Chamaecyparis obtusa) Leaf Oil," *Journal of Physiological Anthropology* 34 (2015): 44.

25. Sowndhararajan and Kim, "Influence of Fragrances on Human Psychophysiological Activity."

26. W. Kim et al., "The Effect of Cognitive Behavior Therapy–Based Psychotherapy Applied in a Forest Environment on Physiological Changes and Remission of Major Depressive Disorder," *Psychiatry Investig.* 6, no. 4 (December 2009): 245–54.

27. D. T. C. Cox et al., "Doses of Nearby Nature Simultaneously Associated with Multiple Health Benefits," *Int. J. Environ. Res. Public Health* 14, no. 2 (February 2017): 172.

28. C. A. Capaldi, R. L. Dopko, and J. M. Zelenski, "The Relationship Between Nature Connectedness and Happiness: A Meta-Analysis," *Front. Psychol.* 5 (September 2014): 976.

29. G. MacKerron and S. Mourato, "Happiness Is Greater in Natural Environments," *Glob. Environ. Change* 23, no. 5 (October 2013): 992–1000.

30. For more about Dr. Rhonda Patrick's work, see FoundMyFitness.com.

31. P. K. Piff et al., "Awe, the Small Self, and Prosocial Behavior," *J. Pers. Soc. Psychol.* 108, no. 6 (June 2015): 883–99.

32. M. Rudd, K. D. Vohs, and J. Aaker, "Awe Expands People's Perception of Time, Alters Decision Making, and Enhances Well-Being," *Psychol. Sci.* 23, no. 10 (October 2012): 1130–36.

33. J. W. Zhang et al., "An Occasion for Unselfing: Beautiful Nature Leads to Prosociality," *J. Environ. Psychol.* 37 (March 2014): 61–72.

34. G. Kim et al., "Functional Neuroanatomy Associated with Natural and Urban Scenic Views in the Human Brain: 3.0T Functional MR Imaging," *Korean J. Radiol.* 11, no. 5 (September–October 2010): 507–13.

35. Y. T. Uhls et al., "Five Days at Outdoor Education Camp Without Screens Improves Preteen Skills with Nonverbal Emotion Cues," *Comput. Human Behav.* 39 (October 2014): 387–92.

36. T. Baumgartner et al., "Frequency of Everyday Pro-Environmental Behaviour Is Explained by Baseline Activation in Lateral Prefrontal Cortex," *Sci. Rep.* 9, no. 9 (January 2019).

37. G. X. Mao et al., "Effects of Short-Term Forest Bathing on Human Health in a Broad-Leaved Evergreen Forest in Zhejiang Province, China," *Biomed. Environ. Sci.* 25, no. 3 (June 2012): 317–24.

38. R. A. Atchley, D. L. Strayer, and P. Atchley, "Creativity in the Wild: Improving Creative Reasoning Through Immersion in Natural Settings," *PLoS One* 7, no. 12 (December 2012): e51474.

39. R. Mitchell and F. Popham, "Effect of Exposure to Natural Environ-

ment on Health Inequalities: An Observational Population Study," *Lancet* 372, no. 9650 (November 2008): 1655–60.

40. D. L. Crouse et al., "Urban Greenness and Mortality in Canada's Largest Cities: A National Cohort Study," *Lancet Planet. Health* 1, no. 7 (October 2017): e289–97.

41. D. Vienneau et al., "More Than Clean Air and Tranquillity: Residential Green Is Independently Associated with Decreasing Mortality," *Environ. Int.* 108 (November 2017): 176–84.

42. M. van den Berg et al., "Health Benefits of Green Spaces in the Living Environment: A Systematic Review of Epidemiological Studies," *Urban For. Urban Green.* 14, no. 4 (August 2015): 806–16.

Chapter 7

1. R. H. Lustig, "Processed Food—An Experiment That Failed," *JAMA Pediatr.* 171, no. 3 (March 2017): 212–14.

2. L. Schnabel et al., "Association Between Ultraprocessed Food Consumption and Risk of Mortality Among Middle-Aged Adults in France," *JAMA Intern. Med.* 179, no. 4 (February 2019): 490–98.

3. GBD 2017 Diet Collaborators, "Health Effects of Dietary Risks in 195 Countries, 1990–2017: A Systematic Analysis for the Global Burden of Disease Study 2017," *Lancet* 393, no. 10184 (May 2019): 1958–72.

4. US Department of Health and Human Services, "What Is a Food Additive?," https://www.hhs.gov/answers/public-health-and-safety/what-is-a-food-additive/index.html.

5. US Food and Drug Administration, "Overview of Food Ingredients, Additives & Colors," https://www.fda.gov/food/food-ingredients-packaging/overview-food-ingredients-additives-colors.

6. US Food and Drug Administration, "Overview of Food Ingredients."

7. B. Popkin and C. Hawkes, "The Sweetening of the Global Diet, Particularly Beverages: Patterns, Trends and Policy Responses for Diabetes Prevention," *Lancet Diabetes Endocrinol.* 4, no. 2 (February 2016): 174–86.

8. V. S. Malik et al., "Long-Term Consumption of Sugar-Sweetened and Artificially Sweetened Beverages and Risk of Mortality in US Adults," *Circulation* 139, no. 18 (April 2019): 2113–25.

9. A. Mummert et al., "Stature and Robusticity During the Agricultural Transition: Evidence from the Bioarchaeological Record," *Econ. Hum. Biol.* 9, no. 3 (July 2011): 284–301.

10. Jared Diamond, "The Worst Mistake in the History of the Human Race," *Discover,* May 1987.

11. Diamond, "The Worst Mistake."

12. Yuval Noah Harari, *Sapiens: A Brief History of Humankind* (New York: Harper, 2015).

13. J. Graham Ruby et al., "Estimates of the Heritability of Human Longevity Are Substantially Inflated Due to Assortative Mating," *Genetics* 210, no. 3 (November 1, 2018): 1109–1124.

14. F. N. Jacka et al., "Western Diet Is Associated with a Smaller Hippocampus: A Longitudinal Investigation," *BMC Med.* 13 (September 2015): 215; see also T. Akbaraly et al., "Association of Long-Term Diet Quality with Hippocampal Volume: Longitudinal Cohort Study," *Am. J. Med.* 131, no. 11 (November 2018): 1372–81.

15. A. Ramirez et al., "Elevated HbA1c Is Associated with Increased Risk of Incident Dementia in Primary Care Patients," *J. Alzheimers Dis.* 44, no. 4 (2015): 1203–12.

16. Lustig, "Processed Food."

17. Y. Lee et al., "Cost-Effectiveness of Financial Incentives for Improving Diet and Health through Medicare and Medicaid: A Microsimulation Study," *PLoS Med.* 16, no. 3 (March 2019): e1002761.

18. M. K. Potvin and A. Wanless, "The Influence of the Children's Food and Beverage Advertising Initiative: Change in Children's Exposure to Food Advertising on Television in Canada between 2006–2009," *Int. J. Obes. (Lond.)* 38, no. 4 (April 2014): 558–62.

19. S. Rincón-Gallardo Patiño et al., "Nutritional Quality of Foods and Non-Alcoholic Beverages Advertised on Mexican Television According to Three Nutrient Profile Models," *BMC Public Health* 16 (August 2016): 733.

20. M. M. Romero-Fernández, M. Á. Royo-Bordonada, and F. Rodríguez-Artalejo, "Evaluation of Food and Beverage Television Advertising During Children's Viewing Time in Spain Using the UK Nutrient Profile Model," *Public Health Nutr.* 16, no. 7 (July 2013): 1314–20.

21. M. Hajizadehoghaz, M. Amini, and A. Abdollahi, "Iranian Television

Advertisement and Children's Food Preferences," *Int. J. Prev. Med.* 7 (December 2016): 128.

22. J. L. Harris, J. A. Bargh, and K. D. Brownell, "Priming Effects of Television Food Advertising on Eating Behavior," *Health Psychol.* 28, no. 4 (July 2009): 404–13.

23. E. J. Boyland et al., "Food Choice and Overconsumption: Effect of a Premium Sports Celebrity Endorser," *J. Pediatr.* 163, no. 2 (August 2013): 339–43.

24. J. A. Emond et al., "Exposure to Child-Directed TV Advertising and Preschoolers' Intake of Advertised Cereals," *Am. J. Prev. Med.* 56, no. 2 (2019): e35–e43.

25. M. A. Bragg et al., "Sports Sponsorships of Food and Nonalcoholic Beverages," *Pediatrics* 141, no. 4 (April 2018): e20172822.

26. S. Luo et al., "Abdominal Fat Is Associated with a Greater Brain Reward Response to High-Calorie Food Cues in Hispanic Women," *Obesity (Silver Spring)* 21, no. 10 (October 2013): 2029–36.

27. Y. Yang et al., "Executive Function Performance in Obesity and Overweight Individuals: A Meta-Analysis and Review," *Neurosci. Biobehav. Rev.* 84 (January 2018): 225–44.

28. N. Mac Giollabhui et al., "Executive Dysfunction in Depression in Adolescence: The Role of Inflammation and Higher Body Mass," *Psychol. Med* (March 2019): 1–9.

29. Giollabhui et al., "Executive Dysfunction."

30. J. A. Bremser and G. G. Gallup, "Mental State Attribution and Body Configuration in Women," *Front. Evol. Neurosci.* 4 (January 2012): 1.

31. B. S. Lennerz et al., "Effects of Dietary Glycemic Index on Brain Regions Related to Reward and Craving in Men," *Am. J. Clin. Nutr.* 98, no. 3 (September 2013): 641–47.

32. R. Chen et al., "Decision Making Deficits in Relation to Food Cues Influence Obesity: A Triadic Neural Model of Problematic Eating," *Front. Psychiatry* 9 (June 2018): 264.

33. M. T. Osborne et al., "Amygdalar Activity Predicts Future Incident Diabetes Independently of Adiposity," *Psychoneuroendocrinology* 100 (February 2019): 32–40.

34. S. C. Staubo et al., "Mediterranean Diet, Micro- and Macronutrients,

and MRI Measures of Cortical Thickness," *Alzheimers Dement.* 13, no. 2 (February 2017): 168–77.

35. A. Molfino et al., "The Role for Dietary Omega-3 Fatty Acids Supplementation in Older Adults," *Nutrients* 6, no. 10 (October 2014): 4058–72.

36. R. K. McNamara et al., "Docosahexaenoic Acid Supplementation Increases Prefrontal Cortex Activation During Sustained Attention in Healthy Boys: A Placebo-Controlled, Dose-Ranging, Functional Magnetic Resonance Imaging Study," *Am. J. Clin. Nutr.* 91, no. 4 (April 2010): 1060–67; see also S. C. Dyall, "Long-Chain Omega-3 Fatty Acids and the Brain: A Review of the Independent and Shared Effects of EPA, DPA, and DHA," *Front. Aging Neurosci.* 7 (April 2015): 52.

37. David Perlmutter, *Brain Maker: The Power of Gut Microbes to Heal and Protect Your Brain for Life* (New York: Little, Brown, 2015).

38. M. K. Wium-Andersen et al., "C-Reactive Protein Levels, Psychological Distress, and Depression in 73, 131 Individuals," *JAMA Psychiatry* 70, no. 2 (2013): 176–184

39. V. Valkanova, K. P. Ebmeier, and C. L. Allan, "CRP, IL-6 and Depression: A Systematic Review and Meta-Analysis of Longitudinal Studies," *J. Affect. Disord.* 150, no. 3 (September 2013): 736–44.

40. A. N. Westover and L. B. Marangell, "A Cross-National Relationship Between Sugar Consumption and Major Depression?," *Depress. Anxiety* 16, no. 3 (2002): 118–20.

41. A. Sanchez-Villegas et al., "Added Sugars and Sugar-Sweetened Beverage Consumption, Dietary Carbohydrate Index and Depression Risk in the Seguimiento Universidad de Navarra (SUN) Project," *Br. J. Nutr.* 119, no. 2 (January 2018): 211–21.

42. J. E. Gangwisch et al., "High Glycemic Index Diet as a Risk Factor for Depression: Analyses from the Women's Health Initiative," *Am. J. Clin. Nutr.* 102, no. 2 (August 2015): 454–63.

43. C. Lassale et al., "Healthy Dietary Indices and Risk of Depressive Outcomes: A Systematic Review and Meta-Analysis of Observational Studies," *Mol. Psychiatry* 24, no. 7 (July 2019): 965–86.

44. Glenda Lindseth, Brian Helland, and Julie Caspers, "The Effects of Dietary Tryptophan on Affective Disorders," *Archives of Psychiatric Nursing* 29, no. 2 (April 2015): 102–107.

45. G. Z. Réus et al., "Kynurenine Pathway Dysfunction in the Pathophys-

iology and Treatment of Depression: Evidences from Animal and Human Studies," *J. Psychiatr. Res.* 68 (September 2015): 316–28.

46. Réus et al., "Kynurenine Pathway Dysfunction."

47. J. Savitz, "Role of Kynurenine Metabolism Pathway Activation in Major Depressive Disorder," *Current Topics in Behavioral Neuroscience* 31 (2017): 249–267.

48. T. B. Meier et al., "Relationship between Neurotoxic Kynurenine Metabolites and Reductions in Right Medial Prefrontal Cortical Thickness in Major Depressive Disorder," *Brain Behav. Immun.* 53 (March 2016): 39–48.

49. Y. Zhou et al., "Cross-Sectional Relationship between Kynurenine Pathway Metabolites and Cognitive Function in Major Depressive Disorder," *Psychoneuroendocrinology* 101 (March 2019): 72–79.

50. J. C. Feiger et al., "Inflammation Is Associated with Decreased Functional Connectivity Within Corticostriatal Reward Circuitry in Depression," *Mol. Psychiatry* 21, no. 10 (October 2016): 1358–65.

51. M. Visser et al., "Elevated C-Reactive Protein Levels in Overweight and Obese Adults," *JAMA* 282, no. 22 (December 1999): 2131–35.

52. K. A. Walker et al., "Midlife Systemic Inflammatory Markers Are Associated with Late-Life Brain Volume: The ARIC Study," *Neurology* 89, no. 22 (November 2017): 2262–70.

53. Masashi Soga, Kevin J. Gaston, and Yuichi Yamaurac, "Gardening Is Beneficial for Health: A Meta-analysis," *Preventative Medicine Reports* 5 (March 2017): 92–99.

Chapter 8

1. Centers for Disease Control and Prevention, "Short Sleep Duration Among U.S. Adults," https://www.cdc.gov/sleep/data_statistics.html.

2. For access to a library of resources and data about sleep, see the National Sleep Foundation's website at SleepFoundation.org.

3. C. S. Möller-Levet et al., "Effects of Insufficient Sleep on Circadian Rhythmicity and Expression Amplitude of the Human Blood Transcriptome," *Proc. Natl. Acad. Sci. USA* 110, no. 12 (March 2013): E1132–41.

4. Matthew Walker, *Why We Sleep: Unlocking the Power of Sleep and Dreams* (New York: Scribner, 2017).

5. J. G. Jenkins and K. M. Dallenbach, "Obliviscence During Sleep and Waking," *Am. J. Psychol.* 35, no. 4 (October 1924): 605–12.

6. A. S. Lim et al., "Sleep Fragmentation and the Risk of Incident Alzheimer's Disease and Cognitive Decline in Older Persons," *Sleep* 36, no. 7 (July 2013): 1027–32.

7. L. K. Barger et al., "Short Sleep Duration, Obstructive Sleep Apnea, Shiftwork, and the Risk of Adverse Cardiovascular Events in Patients After an Acute Coronary Syndrome," *J. Am. Heart Assoc.* 6, no. 10 (October 2017): e006959.

8. C. W. Kim et al., "Sleep Duration and Progression to Diabetes in People with Prediabetes Defined by HbA$_{1c}$ Concentration," *Diabet. Med.* 34, no. 11 (November 2017): 1591–98.

9. M. R. Irwin, R. Olmstead, and J. E. Carroll, "Sleep Disturbance, Sleep Duration, and Inflammation: A Systematic Review and Meta-Analysis of Cohort Studies and Experimental Sleep Deprivation," *Biol. Psychiatry* 80, no. 1 (July 2016): 40.

10. T. B. Meier et al., "Relationship Between Neurotoxic Kynurenine Metabolites and Reductions in Right Medial Prefrontal Cortical Thickness in Major Depressive Disorder," *Brain Behav. Immun.* 53 (March 2016): 39–48.

11. S. M. Greer, A. N. Goldstein, and M. P. Walker, "The Impact of Sleep Deprivation on Food Desire in the Human Brain," *Nat. Commun.* 4 (2013): 2259.

12. M. P. St-Onge et al., "Short Sleep Duration Increases Energy Intakes but Does Not Change Energy Expenditure in Normal-Weight Individuals," *Am. J. Clin. Nutr.* 94, no. 2 (August 2011): 410–16.

13. J. S. Rihm et al., "Sleep Deprivation Selectively Upregulates an Amygdala–Hypothalamic Circuit Involved in Food Reward," *J. Neurosci.* 39, no. 5 (January 2019): 888–99.

14. C. A. Everson, "Functional Consequences of Sustained Sleep Deprivation in the Rat," *Behav. Brain. Res.* 69, nos. 1–2 (July–August 1995): 43–54.

15. J. J. Iliff et al., "A Paravascular Pathway Facilitates CSF Flow Through the Brain Parenchyma and the Clearance of Interstitial Solutes, Including Amyloid β," *Sci. Transl. Med.* 4, no. 147 (August 2012): 147ra111.

16. L. Xie et al., "Sleep Drives Metabolite Clearance from the Adult Brain," *Science* 342, no. 6156 (October 2013): 373–77.

17. E. Shokri-Kojori et al., "β-Amyloid Accumulation in the Human Brain After One Night of Sleep Deprivation," *Proc. Natl. Acad. Sci. USA* 115, no. 17 (April 2018): 4483–88.

18. P. Li et al., "Beta-Amyloid Deposition in Patients with Major Depressive Disorder with Differing Levels of Treatment Resistance: A Pilot Study," *EJNMMI Res.* 7, no. 1 (December 2017): 24; see also S. Perin et al., "Amyloid Burden and Incident Depressive Symptoms in Preclinical Alzheimer's Disease," *J. Affect. Disord.* 229 (March 2018): 269–74.

19. E. Flores-Martinez and F. Peña-Ortega, "Amyloid β Peptide–Induced Changes in Prefrontal Cortex Activity and Its Response to Hippocampal Input," *Int. J. Pept.* 12 (January 2017): 1–9.

20. B. T. Kress et al., "Impairment of Paravascular Clearance Pathways in the Aging Brain," *Ann. Neurol.* 76, no. 6 (December 2014): 845–61.

21. S. Yoo et al., "The Human Emotional Brain Without Sleep—A Prefrontal Amygdala Disconnect," *Curr. Biol.* 17, no. 20 (2007): 877–78.

22. E. van der Helm and M. P. Walker, "Overnight Therapy? The Role of Sleep in Emotional Brain Processing," *Psychol. Bull.* 135, no. 5 (September 2009): 731–48.

23. A. N. Goldstein and M. P. Walker, "The Role of Sleep in Emotional Brain Function," *Annu. Rev. Clin. Psychol.* 10 (2014): 679–708.

24. Y. Motomura et al., "Two Days' Sleep Debt Causes Mood Decline During Resting State via Diminished Amygdala-Prefrontal Connectivity," *Sleep* 40, no. 10 (October 2017).

25. E. Ben Simon and M. P. Walker, "Sleep Loss Causes Social Withdrawal and Loneliness," *Nat. Commun.* 9, no. 3146 (August 2018).

26. K. J. Brower and B. E. Perron, "Sleep Disturbance as a Universal Risk Factor for Relapse in Addictions to Psychoactive Substances," *Med. Hypotheses* 74, no. 5 (May 2010): 928–33.

27. Grand View Research, "Insomnia Therapeutics Market Analysis by Treatment Type [Devices, Drugs (Benzodiazepines, Nonbenzodiazepines, Antidepressants, Orexin Antagonists, Melatonin Antagonists)], by Sales Channel, and Segment Forecasts, 2018–2025," October 2017, https://www.grandviewresearch.com/industry-analysis/insomnia-therapeutics-market.

28. Yinong Chong, Cheryl D. Fryar, and Quiping Gu, "Prescription Sleep Aid Use Among Adults: United States, 2005–2010," Centers for Disease

Control and Prevention, NCHS Data Brief 127, August 2013, https://www.cdc.gov/nchs/products/databriefs/db127.htm.

29. T. B. Huedo-Medina et al., "Effectiveness of Non-Benzodiazepine Hypnotics in Treatment of Adult Insomnia: Meta-Analysis of Data Submitted to the Food and Drug Administration," *BMJ* 345 (December 2012): e8343.

30. D. F. Kripke, R. D. Langer, and L. E. Kline, "Hypnotics' Association with Mortality or Cancer: A Matched Cohort Study," *BMJ Open* 2 (2012): e000850.

31. D. F. Kripke, "Hypnotic Drug Risks of Mortality, Infection, Depression, and Cancer: But Lack of Benefit," version 3, *F1000Res.* 5 (2016): 918.

32. Kripke, "Hypnotic Drug Risks."

33. A. M. Chang et al., "Evening Use of Light-Emitting eReaders Negatively Affects Sleep, Circadian Timing, and Next-Morning Alertness," *Proc. Natl. Acad. Sci. USA* 112, no. 4 (January 2015): 1232–37.

34. J. M. Zeitzer et al., "Sensitivity of the Human Circadian Pacemaker to Nocturnal Light: Melatonin Phase Resetting and Suppression," *J. Physiol.* 526, part 3 (August 2000): 695–702.

35. A. Garcia-Saenz et al., "Evaluating the Association Between Artificial Light-at-Night Exposure and Breast and Prostate Cancer Risk in Spain (MCC-Spain Study)," *Environ. Health Perspect.* 126, no. 4 (April 2018): 047011.

36. P. James et al., "Outdoor Light at Night and Breast Cancer Incidence in the Nurses' Health Study II," *Environ. Health Perspect.* 125, no. 8 (August 2017): 087010.

37. T. A. Bedrosian and R. J. Nelson, "Timing of Light Exposure Affects Mood and Brain Circuits," *Transl. Psychiatry* 7, no. 1 (January 2017): e1017.

38. Common Sense Media, "The Common Sense Census: Media Use by Kids Age Zero to Eight 2017," https://www.commonsensemedia.org/research/the-common-sense-census-media-use-by-kids-age-zero-to-eight-2017.

39. The National Sleep Foundation's Sleep in America poll: https://www.sleepfoundation.org/sites/default/files/inline-files/Highlights_facts_06.pdf.

40. A. Shechter et al., "Blocking Nocturnal Blue Light for Insomnia: A Randomized Controlled Trial," *J. Psychiatr. Res.* 96 (January 2018): 196–202.

41. F. H. Rångtell et al., "Two Hours of Evening Reading on a Self-Luminous Tablet vs. Reading a Physical Book Does Not Alter Sleep After Daytime Bright Light Exposure," *Sleep Med.* 23 (July 2016): 111–18.

Chapter 9

1. D. A. Raichlen and A. D. Gordon, "Relationship Between Exercise Capacity and Brain Size in Mammals," *PLoS One* 6, no. 6 (June 2011): e20601; see also D. A. Raichlen and J. D. Polk, "Linking Brains and Brawn: Exercise and the Evolution of Human Neurobiology," *Proc. Biol. Sci.* 280, no. 1750 (January 2013): 201222550.
2. M. Moriya, C. Aoki, and K. Sakatani, "Effects of Physical Exercise on Working Memory and Prefrontal Cortex Function in Post-Stroke Patients," *Adv. Exp. Med. Biol.* 923 (2016): 203–8; see also T. Tsujii, K. Komatsu, and K. Sakatani, "Acute Effects of Physical Exercise on Prefrontal Cortex Activity in Older Adults: A Functional Near-Infrared Spectroscopy Study," *Adv. Exp. Med. Biol.* 765 (2013): 293–98.
3. S. Dimitrov, E. Hulteng, and S. Hong, "Inflammation and Exercise: Inhibition of Monocytic Intracellular TNF Production by Acute Exercise via β2-Adrenergic Activation," *Brain Behav. Immun.* 61 (March 2016): 60–68.
4. D. Aune et al., "Physical Activity and the Risk of Type 2 Diabetes: A Systematic Review and Dose-Response Meta-Analysis," *Eur. J. Epidemiol.* 30, no. 7 (July 2015): 529–42.
5. E. E. Hill et al., "Exercise and Circulating Cortisol Levels: The Intensity Threshold Effect," *J. Endocrinol. Invest.* 31, no. 7 (July 2008): 587–91.
6. D. E. Lieberman, "Is Exercise Really Medicine? An Evolutionary Perspective," *Curr. Sports Med. Rep.* 14, no. 4 (July–August 2015): 313–19; see also Dr. Lieberman's book *The Story of the Human Body: Evolution, Health, and Disease* (New York: Pantheon, 2013).
7. D. Berrigan et al., "Physical Activity in the United States Measured by Accelerometer," *Med. Sci. Sports Exerc.* 40, no. 1 (January 2008): 181–88.
8. Frank W. Marlowe, *The Hadza: Hunter-Gatherers of Tanzania*, Origins of Human Behavior and Culture 3 (Berkeley: University of California Press, 2010).

9. A. Biswas et al., "Sedentary Time and Its Association with Risk for Disease Incidence, Mortality, and Hospitalization in Adults: A Systematic Review and Meta-Analysis," *Ann. Intern. Med.* 162, no. 2 (January 2015): 123–32.

10. S. Beddhu et al., "Light-Intensity Physical Activities and Mortality in the United States General Population and CKD Subpopulation," *Clin. J. Am. Soc. Nephrol.* 10, no. 7 (July 2015): 1145–53.

11. See the National Cancer Institute's site devoted to covering the relationship between physical activity and cancer: www.cancer.gov/about -cancer/causes-prevention/risk/obesity/physical-activity-fact-sheet.

12. S. Colcombe and A. F. Kramer, "Fitness Effects on the Cognitive Function of Older Adults: A Meta-Analytic Study," *Psychol. Sci.* 14, no. 2 (March 2003): 125–30.

13. C. L. Davis et al., "Exercise Improves Executive Function and Achievement and Alters Brain Activation in Overweight Children: A Randomized, Controlled Trial," *Health Psychol.* 30, no. 1 (January 2011): 91–98.

14. D. Moreau, I. J. Kirk, and K. E. Waldie, "High-Intensity Training Enhances Executive Function in Children in a Randomized, Placebo-Controlled Trial," *Elife* 6 (August 2017).

15. C. E. Hugenschmidt et al., "Effects of Aerobic Exercise on Functional Connectivity of Prefrontal Cortex in MCI: Results of a Randomized Controlled Trial," *Alzheimers Dement.* 13, no. 7 (July 2017): 569–70.

16. J. A. Blumenthal et al., "Lifestyle and Neurocognition in Older Adults with Cognitive Impairments," *Neurology* 92, no. 3 (2019): e212-e223.

17. P. Gellert et al., "Physical Activity Intervention in Older Adults: Does a Participating Partner Make a Difference?," *Eur. J. Ageing* 8, no. 3 (September 2011): 211.

18. A. Kassavou, A. Turner, and D. P. French, "Do Interventions to Promote Walking in Groups Increase Physical Activity? A Meta-Analysis," *Int. J. Behav. Nutr. Phys. Act.* 10 (February 2013) 18.

19. L. Chaddock-Heyman et al., "Aerobic Fitness Is Associated with Greater White Matter Integrity in Children," *Front. Hum. Neurosci.* 8 (August 2014): 584.

20. S. M. Hayes et al., "Cardiorespiratory Fitness Is Associated with White Matter Integrity in Aging," *Ann. Clin. Trans. Neurol.* 2, no. 6 (June 2015): 688–98.

21. C. J. Vesperman et al., "Cardiorespiratory Fitness Attenuates Age-Associated Aggregation of White Matter Hyperintensities in an At-Risk Cohort," *Alzheimers Res. Ther.* 10, no. 1 (September 2018): 97.

22. S. Müller et al., "Relationship Between Physical Activity, Cognition, and Alzheimer Pathology in Autosomal Dominant Alzheimer's Disease," *Alzheimers Dement.* 14, no. 11 (November 2018): 1427–37.

23. Helena Hörder et al., "Midlife Cardiovascular Fitness and Dementia," *Neurology* 90, no. 15 (April 2018): e1298–e1305.

24. G. M. Cooney et al., "Exercise for Depression," *Cochrane Database Syst. Rev.* 9 (September 2013): CD004366.

25. D. Catalan-Matamoros et al., "Exercise Improves Depressive Symptoms in Older Adults: An Umbrella Review of Systematic Reviews and Meta-Analyses," *Psychiatry Res.* 244 (October 2016): 202–9.

26. S. B. Harvey et al., "Exercise and the Prevention of Depression: Results of the HUNT Cohort Study," *Am. J. Psychiatry* 175, no. 1 (January 2017): 28–36.

27. K. W. Choi et al., "Assessment of Bidirectional Relationships Between Physical Activity and Depression Among Adults: A 2-Sample Mendelian Randomization Study," *JAMA Psychiatry* 76, no. 4 (January 2019): 399–408.

28. S. Butscheidt et al., "Impact of Vitamin D in Sports: Does Vitamin D Insufficiency Compromise Athletic Performance?," *Sportverletz Sportschaden* 31, no. 1 (January 2017): 37–44.

Chapter 10

1. S. Charron and E. Koechlin, "Divided Representation of Concurrent Goals in the Human Frontal Lobes," *Science* 328, no. 5976 (April 2010): 360–63.

2. "Use of Yoga and Meditation Becoming More Popular in U.S.," press release, November 8, 2018, https://www.cdc.gov/nchs/pressroom/nchs _press_releases/2018/201811_Yoga_Meditation.htm.

3. P. H. Ponte Márquez et al., "Benefits of Mindfulness Meditation in Reducing Blood Pressure and Stress in Patients with Arterial Hypertension," *J. Hum. Hypertens.* 33, no. 3 (March 2019): 237–47.

4. L. Hilton et al., "Mindfulness Meditation for Chronic Pain: Systematic Review and Meta-Analysis," *Ann. Behav. Med.* 51, no. 2 (April 2017): 199–213.

5. D. S. Black and G. M. Slavich, "Mindfulness Meditation and the Immune System: A Systematic Review of Randomized Controlled Trials," *Ann. N. Y. Acad. Sci.* 1373, no. 1 (June 2016): 13–24.

6. M. C. Pascoe et al., "Mindfulness Mediates the Physiological Markers of Stress: Systematic Review and Meta-Analysis," *J. Psychiatr. Res.* 95 (December 2017): 156–78.

7. T. Gard, B. K. Hölzel, and S. W. Lazar, "The Potential Effects of Meditation on Age-Related Cognitive Decline: A Systematic Review," *Ann. N. Y. Acad. Sci.* 1307 (January 2014): 89–103.

8. J. Ong and D. Sholtes, "A Mindfulness-Based Approach to the Treatment of Insomnia," *J. Clin. Psychol.* 66, no. 11 (November 2010): 1175–84.

9. D. C. Johnson et al., "Modifying Resilience Mechanisms in At-Risk Individuals: A Controlled Study of Mindfulness Training in Marines Preparing for Deployment," *Am. J. Psychiatry* 171, no. 8 (August 2014): 844–53.

10. M. Goyal et al., "Meditation Programs for Psychological Stress and Well-Being: A Systematic Review and Meta-Analysis," *JAMA Intern. Med.* 174, no. 3 (March 2014): 357–68.

11. D. W. Orme-Johnson and V. A. Barnes, "Effects of the Transcendental Meditation Technique on Trait Anxiety: A Meta-Analysis of Randomized Controlled Trials," *J. Altern. Complement. Med.* 20, no. 5 (May 2014): 330–41.

12. B. K. Hölzel et al., "Mindfulness Practice Leads to Increases in Regional Brain Gray Matter Density," *Psychiatry Res.* 191, no. 1 (January 2011): 36–43.

13. S. W. Lazar et al., "Meditation Experience Is Associated with Increased Cortical Thickness," *Neuroreport* 16, no. 17 (November 2005): 1893–97.

14. Y-Y. Tang et al., "Short-Term Meditation Induces White Matter Changes in the Anterior Cingulate," *Proc. Natl. Acad. Sci. USA* 107, no. 35 (2010): 15649–52.

15. J. A. Brewer et al., "Meditation Experience Is Associated with Differences in Default Mode Network Activity and Connectivity," *Proc. Natl. Acad. Sci. USA* 108, no. 50 (December 2011): 20254–59.

16. Y-Y. Tang et al., "Short-Term Meditation Training Improves Attention and Self-Regulation," *Proc. Natl. Acad. Sci. USA* 104, no. 43 (October 2007): 17152–56.

17. Y-Y. Tang, B. K. Hölzel, and M. I. Posner, "The Neuroscience of Mindfulness Meditation," *Nat. Rev. Neurosci.* 16, no. 4 (April 2015): 213–25.

18. S. L. Valk et al., "Structural Plasticity of the Social Brain: Differential Change After Socio-Affective and Cognitive Mental Training," *Sci. Adv.* 3, no. 10 (October 2017): e1700489; see also R. A. Gotink et al., "8-Week Mindfulness Based Stress Reduction Induces Brain Changes Similar to Traditional Long-Term Meditation Practice—A Systematic Review," *Brain Cogn.* 108 (October 2016): 32–41.

19. C. A. Hutcherson, E. M. Seppala, and J. J. Gross, "Loving-kindness Meditation Increases Social Connectedness," *Emotion* 8, no. 5 (October 2008): 720–24.

20. A. A. Taren et al., "Mindfulness Meditation Training and Executive Control Network Resting State Functional Connectivity: A Randomized Controlled Trial," *Psychom. Med.* 79, no. 6 (July–August 2017): 674–83.

21. A. A. Taren, J. D. Creswell, and P. J. Gianaros, "Dispositional Mindfulness Co-Varies with Smaller Amygdala and Caudate Volumes in Community Adults," *PLoS One* 8, no. 5 (May 2013): e64574.

22. G. Desbordes et al., "Effects of Mindful-Attention and Compassion Meditation Training on Amygdala Response to Emotional Stimuli in an Ordinary, Non-Meditative State," *Front. Hum. Neurosci.* 6 (November 2012): 292.

23. C. Wamsler et al., "Mindfulness in Sustainability Science, Practice, and Teaching," *Sustain. Sci.* 13, no. 1 (2018): 143–62.

24. See BensonHenryInstitute.org.

25. M. K. Bhasin et al., "Relaxation Response Induces Temporal Transcriptome Changes in Energy Metabolism, Insulin Secretion and Inflammatory Pathways," *PLoS One* 8, no. 5 (May 2013): e62817.

26. M. De Jong et al., "A Randomized Controlled Pilot Study on Mindfulness-Based Cognitive Therapy for Unipolar Depression in Patients with Chronic Pain," *J. Clin. Psychiatry* 79, no. 1 (January–February 2018): 26–34.

27. J. J. Miller, K. Fletcher, and J. Kabat-Zinn, "Three-Year Follow-Up and

Clinical Implications of a Mindfulness Meditation-Based Stress Reduction Intervention in the Treatment of Anxiety Disorders," *Gen. Hosp. Psychiatry* 17, no. 3 (May 1995): 192–200.

28. To access Dr. Newberg's studies, see http://www.andrewnewberg.com/pdfs.

29. A. B. Newberg et al., "Meditation Effects on Cognitive Function and Cerebral Blood Flow in Subjects with Memory Loss: A Preliminary Study," *J. Alzheimers Dis.* 20, no. 2 (2010): 517–26.

30. A. S. Moss et al., "Effects of an 8-Week Meditation Program on Mood and Anxiety in Patients with Memory Loss," *J. Altern. Complement. Med.* 18, no. 1 (January 2012): 48–53.

31. I. Kirste et al., "Is Silence Golden? Effects of Auditory Stimuli and Their Absence on Adult Hippocampal Neurogenesis," *Brain Struct. Funct.* 220, no. 2 (March 2015): 1221–28.

32. L. Bernardi, C. Porta, and P. Sleight, "Cardiovascular, Cerebrovascular, and Respiratory Changes Induced by Different Types of Music in Musicians and Non-Musicians: The Importance of Silence," *Heart* 92, no. 4 (2006): 445–52.

Chapter 11

1. G. Y. Kim, D. Wang, and P. Hill, "An Investigation into the Multifaceted Relationship Between Gratitude, Empathy, and Compassion," *J. Posit. Psychol. Wellbeing* 2, no. 1 (2018): 23–44.

Conclusion

1. See AdultDevelopmentStudy.org.

2. R. J. Waldinger et al., "Security of Attachment to Spouses in Late Life: Concurrent and Prospective Links with Cognitive and Emotional Well-Being," *Clin. Psychol. Sci.* 3, no. 4 (July 2015): 516–29.

3. John Bowlby, *Attachment and Loss,* vol. 1, *Attachment* (New York: Basic Books, 1969).

4. R. J. Waldinger, G. E. Vaillant, and E. J. Orav, "Childhood Sibling Relationships as a Predictor of Major Depression in Adulthood: A

30-Year Prospective Study," *Am. J. Psychiatry* 164, no. 6 (June 2007): 949–54.

5. Y. Minagawa and Y. Saito, "Active Social Participation and Mortality Risk Among Older People in Japan: Results from a Nationally Representative Sample," *Res. Aging* 37, no. 5 (July 2015): 481–99.

6. S. Cohen et al., "Social Ties and Susceptibility to the Common Cold," *JAMA* 277, no. 24 (June 1997): 1940–44.

7. K. Orth-Gomér, A. Rosengren, and L. Wilhelmsen, "Lack of Social Support and Incidence of Coronary Heart Disease in Middle-Aged Swedish Men," *Psychosom. Med.* 55, no. 1 (January–February 1993): 37–43.

8. See BlueZones.com.

About the Authors

DAVID PERLMUTTER, MD, is a board-certified neurologist and fellow of the American College of Nutrition. He is a frequent lecturer at symposia sponsored by institutions such as the World Bank, Columbia University, New York University, Yale University, and Harvard University and serves as an associate professor at the University of Miami Miller School of Medicine. He is the recipient of numerous awards, including the Linus Pauling Award for his innovative approaches to neurological disorders, the National Nutritional Foods Association Clinician of the Year Award, and the Humanitarian Award from the American College of Nutrition. He maintains an active blog at DrPerlmutter.com and is the author of *Grain Brain, Brain Maker, The Grain Brain Whole Life Plan, The Grain Brain Cookbook,* and *Raise a Smarter Child by Kindergarten.*

AUSTIN PERLMUTTER, MD, is a board-certified internal medicine physician. He received his medical degree from the University of Miami and completed his internal medicine residency at Oregon Health & Science University, in Portland, Oregon. His academic interests center on studying the effects of burnout and depression as well as preventive care and chronic disease management.